QUALITY ASSURANCE
An Introduction for Health Care Professionals

For Churchill Livingstone
Publisher: Mary Law
Project Editor: Dinah Thom
Editorial Co-ordination: Editorial Resources Unit
Production Controller: Nancy Henry
Design: Design Resources Unit
Sales Promotion Executive: Hilary Brown

QUALITY ASSURANCE
An Introduction for Health Care Professionals

Project Co-ordinators

Christine C. Wright BSc AFIMA FSS

Senior Lecturer in Statistics, Department of Statistics and Operational Research, Coventry Polytechnic

Dorothy Whittington MA MEd TCert AFBPsS CPsychol

Director, Centre for Health and Social Research, University of Ulster

Project Team (Ulster)

Hugh McKenna RPN SRN DipN (London) BSc(Hons) RNT

Lecturer in Nursing, Department of Nursing Studies, University of Ulster

Project Team (Coventry)

Lorraine H. Ingleston MA BSc RGN DipN(London) CertEd RNT

Head of Development and Research (now Head of Quality and Resource Management),
United Midlands College for Nursing and Midwifery

Ann P. Moore PhD Grad Dip Phys MCSP DipTP Cert Ed

Senior Lecturer in Physiotherapy, Department of Health Sciences, Coventry Polytechnic
(now Principal Lecturer in Physiotherapy, Brighton Polytechnic)

Karen Ward DipCOT SROT BSc

Lecturer in Occupational Therapy, Department of Health Sciences, Coventry Polytechnic

Foreword by

Norma G. Reid BSc MSc DPhil FSS

Chair of Faculty of Social, Biological and Health Sciences, Coventry Polytechnic

Roger Ellis BA TCert CPsychol AFBPsS

Dean of the Faculty of Social and Health Sciences, University of Ulster

CHURCHILL LIVINGSTONE
EDINBURGH LONDON MADRID MELBOURNE NEW YORK AND TOKYO 1992

CHURCHILL LIVINGSTONE
Medical Division of Longman Group UK Limited

Distributed in the United States of America by Churchill
Livingstone Inc., 650 Avenue of the Americas, New York, N.Y. 10011,
and by associated companies, branches and representatives
throughout the world.

First published 1992

ISBN 0-443-04681-6

British Library Cataloguing in Publication Data
A catalogue record for this book is available from the British
Library.

Library of Congress Cataloging in Publication Data
A catalog record for this book is available from the Library of
Congress.

The
publisher's
policy is to use
**paper manufactured
from sustainable forests**

Produced by Longman Singapore Publishers Pte Ltd
Printed in Singapore

Foreword

The assurance of quality is fundamental to the delivery of health care. Whilst health professionals, individually and collectively, have always placed great importance on the provision of high quality care, it is now recognised that the assurance of quality requires a systematised explicit management strategy which is constantly evaluated and refined.

Quality assurance has a contribution to make to every facet of health care organisation, planning and delivery. Its role has become central in the evaluation of treatment, in the facilitation of purchaser and provider relationships and in establishing that value for money is being sought and obtained. Its role in the organisation and management of health care services is self-evident. But quality assurance is not just a valuable tool for those who manage or plan; it is an essential part of the day-to-day skills of every health care practitioner who directly cares for a patient or client.

It follows that the skills of quality assurance should be taught within the initial educational courses for the health care professions and, indeed, many educational institutions now include quality assurance within their curriculum. In our work we have become aware of the dearth of suitable texts for students. The timely advent of this self-instructional text, designed for students of the health care professions, will enable widespread adoption of the principles of quality assurance within courses, and will also be invaluable to individual users new to this subject area.

We commend this workbook for its user-friendliness, its lucidity and its eclectic approach to the use of quality assurance in health care. The writing team benefits from its interprofessional and interdisciplinary composition, encompassing nursing, physiotherapy, occupational therapy, statistics and psychology. The experience of the team includes the application of quality assurance in industry and in health care settings.

The workbook provides a wealth of practical strategies for the health care practitioner to apply in everyday working conditions. It enables the reader to work at his or her own pace and to adapt the material to his or her own health care practice. We hope and expect that those who use this text will enjoy it, will learn from it and will as a result be able to provide even better care for patients and clients.

N.G.R.
R.E.

Acknowledgements

The authors wish to acknowledge and thank all those who have assisted in the development of this workbook. In particular, we wish to thank Professor Norma Reid and Professor Roger Ellis for their foresight and creativity in the early genesis of the project and for their continuing support; Professor Jenny Boore, Mr Roger Braithwaite and Mrs Margaret Crotty for their support throughout the project; Mrs Louise Poole for her assistance with reference material at an early stage; Mr Rob Solomon for his advice on self-instructional learning materials; Mr Mike Hewitt and Mr Clive Dixon of the Teaching Resources Unit of Coventry Polytechnic for cartoon illustrations, advice on layout and for the painstaking production of the camera-ready copy. Special thanks are also extended to the students who worked through early versions of the workbook, and to the reveiwers who, by their constructive comments, helped the authors keep the customers' viewpoint clearly in focus.

C.C.W.
D.W.

Contents

Unit Three FOLLOWING THE STEPS

Unit Four LOOKING TO THE FUTURE

Introduction to the Workbook

Welcome to this workbook. It is written for readers who wish to investigate the basic concepts of quality assurance. It is suitable for pre- and post-registration health care professionals who have a knowledge of clinical practice, and for social workers.

The aims for this workbook are:

❑ to provide an overview of quality assurance for you, the health care professional;
❑ to sketch the historical background to quality assurance development;
❑ to increase your understanding and appreciation of quality assurance in your professional field;
❑ to encourage your enthusiastic participation in quality assurance programmes;
❑ to introduce some quality assurance techniques appropriate to your professional work as a member of a multi-disciplinary team.

To begin with, it will be useful to consider why you are studying this workbook.

✎ Jot down what you hope to have achieved when you have finished studying this workbook.

Individual/group learning

The workbook is designed so that you can study independently, at your own pace. Alternatively, you may choose to work through the book as a member of a group. You might find it easier and more effective to study in short, regular spells. Whichever way you study, you will be encouraged to apply basic concepts to your own working environment and professional practice. You will also be guided towards an interprofessional approach to quality assurance.

Units and Sections

There are four units in the workbook:-

Unit One	:	Understanding Quality
Unit Two	:	Assessing and Improving Quality
Unit Three	:	Following the Steps
Unit Four	:	Looking to the Future

Unit one is written for individuals with little or no prior knowledge of quality assurance. Several sections investigate quality: discussing its meaning, whose business it is, how it is judged and who sets the standards. Further sections present an overview of quality assurance in health care: discussing its meaning, its importance, its evolution and its costs.

Unit two is slightly more technical. It is written for individuals who have studied unit one or who already have a general understanding of quality assurance. It describes how you can take part in quality assurance in your own professional practice and guides you through the necessary stages of quality appraisal and quality action.

Unit three gives you an opportunity to practise some of the techniques that you meet in unit two. A clinical scenario is presented and you are invited to write a standard and related criteria.

Unit four reviews the aims of the workbook and makes suggestions for future work.

Unit one should take about	2-3 hours to complete;
unit two	2-5 hours to complete;
unit three	2-5 hours' activity.

Objectives

Each section begins with a list of **objectives**. These identify the progress you should expect to have made after completing the section.

Activities

To help you achieve the objectives, most sections contain **activities**. These are clearly identified in the text. A pen symbol ✎ is used to indicate when you need to make a written response.

An activity requires you to perform some task. It might ask you to:-
- think about a particular idea;
- jot down your opinions or comments upon a particular situation;
- seek information from your workplace;
- critically evaluate given material;
- produce and appraise standards and criteria.

Don't worry if you are uncertain about your responses. We have included brief comments after most of the activities to help you. As this is only an introduction to the subject, these comments are not exhaustive. You may be able to think of additional comments related to your own work area or experience. This will be especially true if you are working in a group where you will be sharing ideas with others and generating lots of discussions and new ideas.

The activities in unit one will each take you   2-10 minutes;
                unit two   2-20 minutes;
                unit three   2-30 minutes.

Self-assessment Questions

Self-assessment questions appear periodically in the workbook. The questions should only take a few minutes to answer and will help you to chart your progress. Solutions are given immediately after the questions.

References

A short list of supportive reading material and references are given at the end of the workbook. We hope you will find this useful.

Glossary

We have included a glossary of important terms so that, if necessary, you can check their meanings.

A Message from the Authors

We hope that you will find this workbook informative and instructional, as well as enjoyable and intellectually stimulating.

Now read on.

Unit One

UNDERSTANDING QUALITY

6

1 Introduction to Understanding Quality

> **Objective**
> By the end of this section you will be able to:
> ● describe quality and quality assurance in your own terms.

Quality is a word that is commonly used both in the work environment and in the home setting. But as a concept quality is hard to define. We begin by asking you questions about your existing knowledge. At the end of the unit, you will be asked to review your answers.

✎[a] Jot down what you understand by the term quality.

On a scale of 1 (low confidence) to 5 (high confidence) mark how confident you are about this:

scale 1 2 3 4 5

✎[b] You may have met the term 'quality assurance'. What do you think it means?

As above, on a scale of 1 (low confidence) to 5 (high confidence) mark how confident you are about this:

scale 1 2 3 4 5

✎[c] Have you come across 'quality assurance' in your professional setting? If you have, make a few notes on your experience and list any specific techniques which were used.

✎ [d] If known, say who instigated the quality assurance initiative in your professional workplace.

Now that you have described your understanding of the term quality, let's explore this further.

2 Quality

To help you understand quality consider the following questions:

What is quality?
Whose business is quality?
How is quality judged?
Who sets the standards?

2.1 What is quality?

To help you achieve these objectives, think about some everyday objects such as apples and cars. These will form a useful introduction to the concepts applied later to the health care setting.

Activity
When buying items of food you make decisions about the quality of the food available. Think about buying something as commonplace as an apple.

How do you decide what apple to buy?

✎ Here are some characteristics that might be important. Put a tick against any that you would consider before buying an apple. Add any other characteristics that would influence your purchase.

looks	____
colour	____
variety	____
size	____
smell	____
firmness	____
texture	____
taste	____
country of origin	____
other (please specify)	____

✎ Use this information to produce your definition of a quality apple.

✎ Do you think that everyone will produce the same definition, that is, aim to buy the same apple? Give reasons for your answer.

Obviously, people have different tastes and one person's opinion of what constitutes a quality apple (for example, shiny red skin, juicy, crisp, sweet, English, no blemishes...) may be unacceptable to another person. Many features go to make up quality and people interpret quality in different ways. However, in your definition you probably assumed an intended use for the apple. Was it to be eaten with your lunch, or was it to be cooked in an apple pie? Your view of a quality apple would differ in these two situations. For example, you might accept a small blemish on a cooking apple, but not on an eating apple. Further, you have probably added cost to the list of characteristics. You want an apple with features that you think are suitable for your intended use and at the right price. This represents one view of quality.

Activity
Let's pursue this view with a manufactured product, a car.
Consider the following two situations:

A)   You are a family person, with a spouse and two children. You own a family car. You want a second car solely to transport you the short distance between home and work.

B)   You are a successful business person. You want a car to impress potential customers.

✎ For each situation, jot down a list of features that in your opinion characterises a quality car.
In situation A, a car needs to be ...

✎ In situation B, a car needs to be ...

Features that could appear in your specification of a quality car include–reliability, safety, durability, purchase cost, running costs, maintenance costs, engine performance, styling, colour, comfort, quietness, size, age, luxury of interior, accessories and extras.

In situation A, the second car needs to be reasonably priced, fairly quiet and comfortable, cheap to run, service and maintain, and acceptable in looks. In situation B, the business person's car needs to be expensive, luxurious, comfortable, powerful, quiet, stylish and reliable. The latter description is a commonly held view of a quality car. It implies a grading on each feature, with high quality equating with high grade and, usually, high cost. This ignores the intended use of the car. It means that a small, basic car cannot be regarded as a quality product even if it is superbly designed and manufactured, never breaks down and is very cheap to run, service and maintain. However, if quality is taken as suitability for intended use at an acceptable cost, then such a car could be rated comparable in quality with a Rolls Royce.

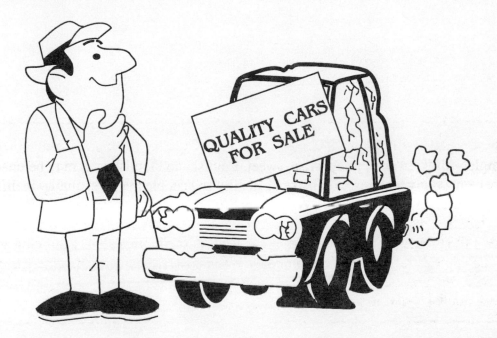

The examples we used of an apple and a car have shown that it is quite easy to list features that describe the quality of a given product. It is more difficult to describe quality in relation to health care. Health care is a mix of services ranging from health promotion to organ transplantation.

Quality of care involves both the technical aspects of providing services and the human aspects which arise from the personal contact between the supplier and receiver of care. These personal interactions influence judgements about the quality of care provided and received.

Activity

Let's consider a different example, the professional practitioner. In your own professional field there are some practitioners you admire for the quality of their work. Think of a member of your own profession, a colleague perhaps, who epitomises your concept of a quality professional.

✎ Jot down a list of the attributes which led you to select this person.

Once again, you've produced your view on the attributes of quality in a given situation. These attributes are influenced by your professional background, area of work, status, work environment and so on.

Probably you used words like:

> **C**ommitted, caring, communicative
>
> **A**ccountable, autonomous, approachable
>
> **R**eliable, respected, resourceful
>
> **E**xpert, efficient, ethical

These traits describe someone's ability as a competent practitioner, but they do not describe the service that is provided. The following are some features that you might include if you were asked to describe a quality service in your own area of expertise:

> **C**omprehensive, cost-effective, contractual
>
> **A**ccessible, accredited, acceptable
>
> **R**elevant, reliable, resourced
>
> **E**fficient, equitable, effective

Activity

✎ In the context of your own profession, select one of the personal traits listed above and write down a definition of this trait.

✎ Repeat the exercise for one feature of a quality service from the list above.

If time allows, you may wish to consider some of the other items before you read on.

Note how the definition and priority of each is dependent upon work environment and clinical speciality.

In this section you have considered quality as being suitable for intended use, and listed some features that describe quality. This leads us to question whose business quality is and to ask how it is judged.

2.2 Whose business is quality?

Objectives
By the end of this section you will be able to:
- identify who is interested in quality;
- identify what affects quality;
- discuss who should take responsibility for quality.

Returning to the apple example discussed in the previous section, it is appropriate to consider who is interested in the quality of an apple. Perhaps you will begin by saying that as the consumer you are the only person concerned. But there will be others who will be interested in the quality of an apple on sale. These include the retailer, the wholesaler, distributor and grower. Each person in the chain has an interest in providing a quality apple to you the consumer or end client. Note that some people act both as a customer and a supplier e.g. the retailer. In the health service, the customer and supplier may be called the purchaser and the provider, respectively.

Diagram 1.   Quality Chain

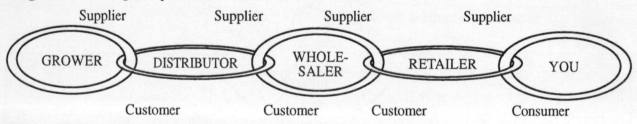

The situation is even more complex in the context of health service and care, as we have seen. The client is the end customer for whom all members of the health care team work together to provide a quality service. It is important to remember that within the team each individual practitioner may be a customer of other members. For example, when a nurse dresses a wound the nurse uses the products of the central sterilisation department and is therefore their customer. Quality in the sterilisation department will affect the quality of care given to the client whose wound is being dressed. The client would be at risk from infection if the dressings were not sterile.

Activity
✎ Take one of your common practice areas and jot down all your customers and suppliers for this area.

You may be able to identify points in the chain where problems or conflicts occur and to recognise how these could affect the quality of care. Conflicts may occur through an inadequate supply of materials, lack of technical equipment, unsuitable treatment rooms, insufficient support staff. Some questions naturally follow such a statement. These include: who judges the degree of inadequacy? ... what is adequate? what is acceptable? .... These are addressed in the next section. Here, it is noted that it is easy to blame problems on the lack of resources. Without doubt, some quality problems can be attributed to this but not all. This too will be discussed later.

Let's return to the question 'whose business is quality?'.
In health care quality involves the inter-relationships between numerous groups of professional and lay people. A simplified view of this relationship is given below:-

Diagram 2.   The Quality Focus

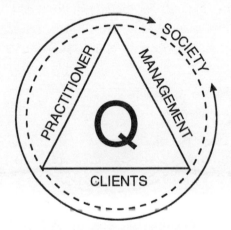

Quality is shown as the central focus of attention for practitioners, managers and clients. Society at large influences the relationships between the groups.

Activity

✎ Consider one of your recent clients, and jot down a list of all the people who could influence the quality of care received by this client.

A wide range of individuals directly and indirectly associated with a client could influence the quality of care. You have probably included in your list the professionals, who provide care on an individual basis, and those whose work is essential in the provision of an overall quality service; for example, catering, cleaning, portering, clerical and administrative staff. If we add the family, community agencies and local pressure groups we can see the size of the network that affects the quality of care for a client.

The following diagram shows some of the individuals and groups who have an interest in the achievement of a quality service. Perhaps you have included some of these in your list.

Diagram 3.   Achieving Quality Care

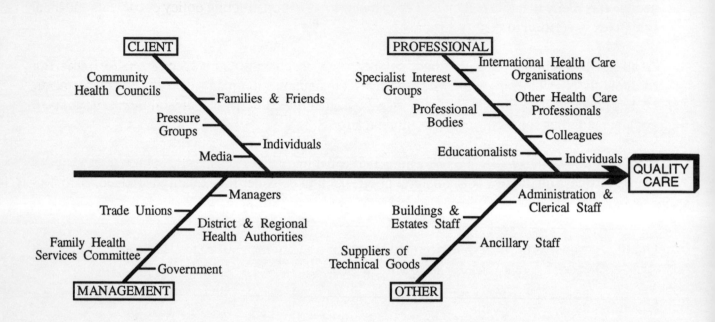

Diagram 3 shows a complex and interactive framework. It illustrates the idea that quality of care is important to clients, practitioners, management and health organisations, and to society as a whole. These groups may be interested in quality for different reasons, will have different perspectives on quality and consequently have different priorities. Their interests may be purely client-centred, or influenced by external pressures such as government policy, scarcity of resources or changing technology.

At an individual level, everyone affects quality of care–receptionists, telephonists, building maintenance staff, managers, clerical staff, caterers, professional staff. **Quality is everyone's business**. There is a potential problem here–since quality is everyone's business it can become no-one's business. Therefore, in any organisation or business, someone needs to take the responsibility for quality. Many Health Authorities have designated a single officer to have overall responsibility. This helps to ensure that quality matters are considered and are taken seriously.

Activity

✎ Identify a senior person with overall responsibility for quality in your workplace.

Perhaps this person is a member of the management board or a senior member of your professional group. It is likely that this person will be in the process of constructing policy documents and local initiatives in relation to quality assurance.

At all levels, it is important to nominate people to have responsibility for specific quality issues. For example, the physiotherapy helper is responsible for maintaining the quality of treatment environments, i.e. bed linen, cleanliness of the hydrotherapy pool. Identified quality responsibilities need to be well documented, thus supporting good communication.

In this section you have discovered who is interested in quality, what could influence quality and whose business quality is. It is a natural progression to consider how quality is judged.

2.3 How is quality judged?

Objectives
After working through this section you will:
- be able to discuss how quality is judged;
- have an awareness of the role of standards and criteria.

In the apple illustration you listed features that in your opinion described a quality apple. Your aim was to buy an apple that satisfied your requirements against each of those features. For example, you determined what colour variation, what range of size, what variety and what price range were acceptable to you. That is, you judged the quality of an apple for an intended use against your pre-determined standards.

In health care too, quality is judged against standards.

Activity

✎ Jot down what you understand by the term 'standard'.

Here is the College of Occupational Therapists' definition:-
'A standard is an acceptable or approved example or statement of something against which measurement and/or judgement takes place; a level of quality relevant to the activity.'

There are several important points in this definition. A standard:-
- ❑ specifies what is important to achieve;
- ❑ specifies levels that have to be achieved;
- ❑ may apply to any activity or feature that is important for quality;
- ❑ may apply to a series of activities or a collection of features that are important for quality.

Here's an example of a standard: '95% of clients at an outpatients' clinic are seen by the consultant no later than 20 minutes after their scheduled appointment time.' Actual achieved performance is measured against identified quality criteria. This is used to judge whether the standard is being met. If in our example records show that 30% of clients wait longer than 20 minutes after their scheduled appointment, then the standard is not being met. Managers can deal with this situation in at least two ways. Changes could be implemented in the service to enable the standard to be met; that is, the quality of service could be improved. For example, the appointments' procedure might be altered. Or it may be decided that the target is unachievable within existing resource availability and the standard changed.

Various frameworks can be used in describing quality. In an early attempt to measure health care quality, Donabedian (1966) proposed three categories into which service could be characterised— structure, process and outcome:-

❑ structure
  –includes personnel, equipment, buildings, record systems, finance, supplies and
    facilities;
❑ process
  –incorporates all aspects of the performance of activities of care;
❑ outcome
  –denotes the end results of care/service.

All three categories need to be considered to obtain a balanced view of quality. For example, it does not automatically follow that a quality service will be delivered just because there is a purpose built environment.

Another framework developed for health from a number of industrial and other sources (Juran, 1988; Maxwell, 1984) is:-

❑ timeliness
  –including access, waiting and action time;
❑ information
  –clarification by answering what, why, how, when, who;
❑ technical competence
  –including medical knowledge, skills and expertise; ethics, technology, completeness
    and success of treatment;
❑ personal interaction with practitioner/client
  –including courtesy, respect, bedside manner;
❑ environment
  –including buildings, cleanliness, amenities.

Activity

✎You are visiting your local general practitioner. Against each feature of care shown in the table below give an example of what is important to you as a client and try to specify the level of service that you want to receive.

FEATURE	CLIENT'S VIEW
Timeliness	
–access	
–waiting	
–action	
Information	
Technical Competence	
Personal Interaction	
Environment	

In trying to specify acceptable levels of service you have probably noted that some were easier than others. Queuing time is easy to measure in, say, minutes. Therefore, it is easy to state an acceptable limit on waiting time. What limits did you specify? Measurements of time are said to be objective. Distance, age, weight, mortality rates and number of clients per session are further examples of objective measures. Objective measures can be easily agreed upon and can be compared with each other.

But how do you measure personal interaction? information? environment? This is likely to be subjective or dependent upon personal perception. Health care professionals are working with social scientists to try and produce comparable measures of such features of quality. When quality of care can be expressed through comparable measures, then the client and society can directly compare the services being provided by different institutions. In an open market this should allow the client to make an informed choice about suppliers of care. Competition between establishments should lead to quality improvement.

Activity
Return to the previous activity and put yourself in the role of the general practitioner. The listed features still allow for a useful overview of the service provided, but your expectations are different in this changed role.

Clients, practitioners, managers, health authorities and organisations will have different views on what is important to quality. These different perspectives are dependent upon knowledge, experience and the situation. For example a client who is to have curative high technology surgery may put more value on technical competence than bedside manner; whereas a client who is dying will value empathy and understanding as highly as technical expertise. In isolation, the various interested parties would judge quality on the basis of different standards and different criteria. It is therefore important to consider who sets the standards.

2.4 Who sets the standards?

Objective
After participating in this section you will be able to:
- identify individuals and groups involved in standard setting.

Activity

✎ In earlier sections you have discussed who is interested in quality of care. This included:-

❑ individuals
    –health care professionals   ___
    –health care workers   ___
    –clients and their families   ___
❑ groups
    –practitioners   ___
    –professional bodies   ___
    –local management   ___
    –consumer bodies   ___
    –society   ___
    –politicians   ___
❑ health authorities
    –local level   ___
    –national level   ___
    –international level   ___
❑ others (please specify)   ___

Place a tick against individuals or groups whom you think should be involved in setting standards in health care. Add to the list any groups that you think have been omitted.

We have represented the major interested parties in a jigsaw, diagram 4, implying that appropriate standards are determined if everyone contributes to their formulation.

Diagram 4.   **The Standard Setters**

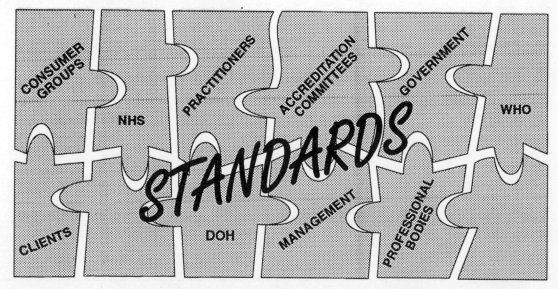

Let's consider some of the categories in more detail.

Every individual who accepts that 'quality is everyone's business' sets personal standards, both in their professional and private roles. These personal standards are informal and are seldom written down or seen by anyone else. Individuals judge their own performance against their own pre-determined specifications. Many judgements will be subjective.

Activity

Ask colleagues from your own discipline how they would describe good professional care.

✎ Jot down a few notes for use in the next activity.

You will probably find some common features across the replies. Many of the features may be difficult to measure objectively.

The client is on the receiving end of care and therefore the client's view of that service is very important. Clients set informal standards on the quality of care that they expect to receive. They can indirectly influence formal standard setting through various consumer bodies and pressure groups. Many studies performed over the last 10 years have investigated clients' subjective opinions. These have enabled clients' views on the quality of care provided to have a direct influence upon formal standards.

Practitioners are involved in setting standards for the care of individual clients. Standards for client care should be set within interprofessional teams–taking an holistic approach to client care. In this way potential conflicts between professional perspectives can be discussed and resolved. Practitioners are also involved in setting standards affecting the quality of the internal service provided.

All of these standards must comply with the standards of care specified by the professional bodies that express their agreed codes of conduct and philosophies of health care.

Activity

Ask colleagues from at least one other discipline how they would describe good professional care. Compare these responses with those from your own discipline. What similarities and differences can you see?

Local management will set standards that specify local commitment to quality and reflect local needs. These standards must be within the framework of standards set by Regional Health Authorities. These in turn are consistent with national standards that define the principles of quality of care.

Activity

Discover what standards have been set by your professional body. If available, select two or three standards. If not, you may like to refer to the examples that follow. Use the following questions to appraise critically each of the standards selected.

1. Does the standard address a clearly defined activity or feature that is important to quality?

2. Does the standard specify:-
   ❑ what is to be achieved;
   ❑ how it is to be achieved;
   ❑ acceptable levels of performance on these criteria.

3. Is there a date for review of the standard?

The outline for these example standards is based on the Dynamic Standard Setting System (DySSSy) (RCN, 1990), which will be discussed in more detail in unit two.

Example Standard 1

Topic: Continuity of care.   **Appraisal date:** 12.6.90
Subtopic: Patient discharge into the community.   **Review date:** 12.12.90
Care Group: All patients on a surgical ward who require   **Authorised by:** S.Smith
continued care in the community.
Standard Statement: All patients understand the care which they require following discharge from hospital, and are visited within 24 hours by a community nurse who administers the referred care.

No.	Structure	No.	Process	No.	Outcome
1	1 referral policy.	1	Nurse explains to patient the care that is required following discharge.	1	Patient can describe the care that is required following discharge.
2	1 liaison sister on duty Mon-Fri (9am-5pm).	2	Nurse explains to patient that community nurse will follow-up care within 24 hours of discharge.	2	Patient receives a visit from community nurse within 24 hours of discharge.
3	Departmental discharge procedure.	3	Nurse in charge of the ward completes the referral form for patient's discharge.	3	Patient receives the referred treatment from the community nurse.
4	All registered nurses have knowledge of discharge procedure.	4	Nurse in charge supplies liaison sister with referral form.		
		5	Nurse in charge of the ward informs liaison sister of the patient's required treatment following discharge.		
		6	Nurse in charge telephones referral directly to community nurse when liaison sister is unavailable.		

Example Standard 2

Topic: Spinal injury.	Appraisal date: 5.2.91
Subtopic: Home assessment prior to discharge from spinal injury unit.	Review date: 5.11.91
Care Group: All clients for whom discharge into a community setting is proposed.	Authorised by: P.Green
Standard Statement: Every client undergoes a comprehensive home assessment, to allow appropriate planning, prior to discharge.	

No.	Structure	No.	Process	No.	Outcome
1	Departmental procedures written on the home assessment process.	1	The occupational therapist identifies the stage at which a home assessment is required within the treatment programme.	1	The client has undergone a comprehensive home assessment.
2	Standardised home assessment documentation.	2	The occupational therapist explains to the client, carers and support services the purpose of the home assessment.	2	The client can describe the care that is required following discharge.
3	Transportation for home assessment available Mon-Fri (9am-5pm).	3	The occupational therapist arranges the date and time of home assessment in consultation with the client, carers and support services.	3	Upon discharge the client is in receipt of the agreed requirements from the home assessment visit.
4	A minimum of 1 qualified occupational therapist and 1 member of support staff available for each home assessment.	4	The occupational therapist performs a detailed daily living and environmental assessment with the client within the proposed home environment.		
		5	The occupational therapist identifies areas where intervention is required to allow maximum independence and safety upon discharge.		
		6	The occupational therapist discusses with the client, carers and the support services methods of over-coming identified problem areas.		
		7	The occupational therapist writes a comprehensive home assessment report detailing requirements prior to discharge.		

Example Standard 3

Topic: Continuity of care.
Subtopic: Client referral.
Care Group: All clients referred for orthopaedic out-patient physiotherapy.
Appraisal date: 31.5.91
Review date: 31.5.92
Authorised by: T.Blue

Standard Statement: Every client has an appointment to attend the out patient department within two weeks of referral.

No.	Structure	No.	Process	No.	Outcome
1	1 receptionist on duty Mon-Fri (8.30am-4.30pm).	1	Receptionist enters client details into departmental records.	1	The client has received an appointment within 2 weeks of the referral date.
2	1 referral policy.	2	The receptionist liaises with the senior physiotherapist.	2	The client's referral has been documented.
3	1 appointment card per client.	3	The senior physiotherapist allocates a therapist to the client.	3	A named physiotherapist has been allocated to the client.
4	1 physiotherapist.	4	The physiotherapist allocates a date for the examination within 2 weeks of referral.		
5	1 senior physiotherapist.	5	The receptionist forwards a completed appointment card to the client.		

You've now completed the first sections of the workbook on Quality. Here are some questions for you to assess your progress.

Self-assessment Question 1

✎ Complete the 'Summary of Quality' by inserting into the spaces provided the eight appropriate words from the list given below.

Wordlist

acceptable	complex	do	grades	satisfying
achieve	criteria	everyone's	important	similar
activities	define	features	levels	simple
any	different	good	no-one's	standards

Summary of Quality

The four questions, 'What is quality?', 'Whose business is quality?', 'How is quality judged?' and 'Who sets the standards?' have been used to give you a general understanding of quality. Through these you should now realise that quality is a _____$_1$ concept. Given a specific need for care, it is possible to list features that describe quality and to list activities that are important to the quality of care. One view of quality is satisfying this specific need at _____$_2$ costs. Satisfaction of the need is judged through pre-determined quality _____$_3$. Standards specify what is important to _____$_4$ and the levels that are required to be achieved.

Actual level of performance of care is measured through criteria specified on the important features and activities. There is a potential problem. Who specifies what is _____$_5$ to quality? People interpret quality in _____$_6$ ways dependent upon, for example, their situation, status, knowledge, environment, interaction with pressure groups and professional bodies.

Clients, managers, practitioners, society and health organisations are all interested in the quality of care and can influence it. Quality is _____$_7$ business. The danger is that it can become _____$_8$ business. Hence, responsibility for quality is assigned to named individuals.

Self-assessment Question 2

✎ Suggest a definition of quality.

Now return to the introduction on page 7 where you first considered quality and compare the two.

Has your understanding changed?

On a scale of 1 (low confidence) to 5 (high confidence) mark how confident you are about your new statement:

scale   1   2   3   4   5

When you have completed this question turn to the glossary and compare your definition.

Self-assessment Question 3

Refer back to the common practice area for which you listed all your customers and suppliers.

✎ i)   What do you think that your customers mean by 'quality'?

ii)   How do you think customers of your service could be made aware of agreed standards and be given an opportunity to comment upon them?

iii)   What standards have you agreed with your suppliers?
        If you have answered 'none', in what priority areas would you first establish standards?

iv)   If you have been unable to answer any of these questions, say why you think this was so.

Self-assessment Question 4

For each of the following statements, decide whether it is true or false.

✎ Circle your answer.
1)   The intended use of a product will affect your opinion about its quality.

                            True/False.

2)   As a health care practitioner, you act as 'supplier' to the client, but you are not a 'customer' of other professionals.

                            True/False.

3)   Although quality is everyone's business, there is a need for a senior manager to take overall responsibility for quality.

                            True/False.

4)   Objective criteria can be measured.

                            True/False.

5)   Height and weight are examples of subjective measures.

                            True/False.

Solutions to self-assessment questions

In many cases these are guidelines to solutions rather than complete answers.

Solution to Self-assessment Question 1

space	word
1	complex
2	acceptable
3	standards
4	achieve
5	important
6	different
7	everyone's
8	no-one's

Solution to Self-assessment Question 2

You will have realised that it is very difficult to write a clear but concise definition of quality. You may have changed your view of quality after working through these sections of the workbook.

Solution to Self-assessment Question 3

There are no unique answers to each part of this question.

i) You may have made a list of some features of your service and some personal characteristics that you think are desirable, similar to our lists on page 13.

ii) You may have suggested documentation of some form, for example contracts, or involvement in joint meetings.

If possible, you could discuss these issues with one of your customers and compare your perceptions with their actual views.

iii) You may find it interesting to discuss this question (indeed all these questions) with peers from both your own and other professional groups.

If you have no agreed standards, you may have suggested giving first consideration according to:
likely adverse effects upon or consequences to your customers;
likely effect on your time;
likely effect on resources.

iv) Now that you have worked through the sections on 'Quality' you may be more aware of the complexity of the issues, but possibly less confident in your understanding. Don't worry, you will become more confident as you proceed through the workbook.

Solution to Self-assessment Question 4

1) True.

The intended use of a product will affect your opinion about its quality; remember our example about the car. You may feel that this is a very obvious statement, but it is nevertheless an important point to make.

2) False.

You form part of a quality chain (like the retailer in our apple example). Perhaps you are a customer of the records department or a pharmacist.

3) True.

We have tried to stress that quality is everyone's business, but that someone needs to be identified to take responsibility. The reason for this should become clearer as you work through the next sections in this unit and through unit two.

Did you manage to identify the senior officer in your workplace with responsibility for quality?

4) True.

Objective criteria can be measured and thereby provide evidence on which to base a judgement about quality. We identified time, distance and mortality rates as examples of objective variables.

5) False.

Height and weight are both examples of objective variables, we can record height in metres and weight in kilograms. In general, it is not easy to record values for subjective variables. We identified perceptions of personal interaction, information and environment as being subjective.

3 Quality Assurance

Objectives

By the end of the sections on Quality Assurance you will be able to:
- suggest a definition for quality assurance;
- report on the importance of quality assurance in health care;
- sketch a background to the development of quality assurance;
- describe the costs associated with quality;
- list some sources of information about quality assurance.

To achieve these objectives you will consider the following questions:-

What is quality assurance?

Why is quality assurance needed in health care?

How has quality assurance evolved in the UK?

What does quality cost?

How do you find out about quality assurance?

3.1 What is quality assurance?

Objective

By the end of this section you will be able to:
- give an overview of quality assurance.

Quality assurance is an integral part of client care activities in all Health Authorities. Its objective is to improve the care provided to clients.

You have seen that quality is a complex concept and elusive to define. It should be no surprise that there is no simple or unique definition of quality assurance.

Activity

✎ Using a dictionary, write down the definition of 'assurance' and the definition of 'assure'.

assurance–

assure–

Your dictionary may have used words such as promise, guarantee and confidence.
How do these relate to the quality of care?

Quality assurance is the effective execution of all the activities concerned with attaining quality. It provides objective evidence that gives clients and society confidence that the quality of care within an institution satisfies stated requirements. This is the level of guarantee.

At a basic level, quality assurance incorporates the following stages (Lang, 1984):
- ❑ setting standards;
- ❑ appraising actual achievements;
- ❑ planning for improvement;
- ❑ taking action when required.

Setting standards involves writing statements that describe achievable and desirable levels of quality of care. These are the professionals' expectations of the service and statement of intent to clients. Appraising actual achievement involves comparing practice with the defined standards through measurement criteria. Any gap between provision and expectation requires action to be taken. This involves planning for improvement. If quality of care is below the stated acceptable levels, then action is taken to raise quality until standards are met.

Quality assurance is a continuous process. Comparison is made periodically which enables the effects of changes to be monitored. If provision is level with or above expectation, then the standard may be changed to specify an improved level of service.

These basic steps are repeated in a cyclical nature, as shown in diagram 5. This is commonly referred to as the quality wheel.

Diagram 5.   A Basic Quality Wheel

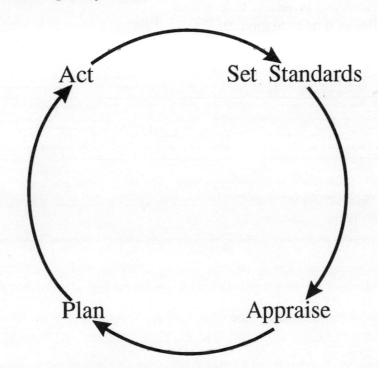

Quality assurance is a never-ending improvement in the quality of care. The basic steps can be viewed as forming a spiral rising to the ultimate quality service. This is shown in diagram 6.

Diagram 6.   Quality Spiral

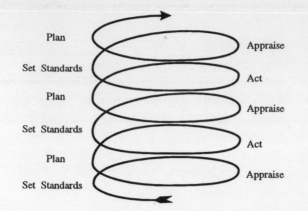

In order to be successful, it is obvious that quality assurance must be organised and managed through a structured system. The coordination of a quality assurance system is the overall responsibility of management. Such a system ensures that quality assurance actually takes place within an organisation and that all associated activities are documented and reported.

Activity

Think about what is needed to support quality assurance initiatives. A list of possible features is given in the table below.

✎ Put a tick against each feature that you think is important in quality assurance.

FEATURE
commitment from top management   _____
commitment from all personnel   _____
clear responsibilities for quality activities   _____
willingness to change   _____
accurate documentation   _____
effective communication at all levels of the organisation   _____
ongoing training programme on quality   _____
ongoing skills training programme   _____

There ought to be ticks against every feature. Clear, detailed and accurate records need to be maintained on procedures to be followed, actions to be taken and actions actually taken.

Effective communication at all levels of the organisation means that people are well informed; that is, the right people have the right information at the right time and in the right place.

Training programmes keep personnel up to date with skills and technical developments. This helps people to perform their duties more effectively and efficiently. Training programmes on quality are important to foster a commitment to quality assurance throughout the organisation. They introduce people to quality techniques that are needed to enable them to take part in quality assurance initiatives.

Top management needs to be committed so that resources are allocated to quality assurance initiatives and actions are followed through. But quality is influenced by everyone, so it is important that all personnel are committed to improvement and are willing to accept and implement change. People need to know what they are expected to do, so responsibilities for quality activities must be clearly assigned.

But why do health care professionals need to change? Indeed, why is quality assurance needed in health care?

3.2 Why is quality assurance needed in health care?

Objective
By the end of this section you will be able to:
● justify the quality assurance programmes in health care.

There are many reasons why quality assurance programmes are needed in health care.

Activity
✎ Consider why you think quality assurance in health care is important, and jot down a few of your ideas.

You may have included points such as accountability, efficiency and economics, as shown in diagram 7.

Diagram 7.   The Incentives for Quality Assurance in Health Care.

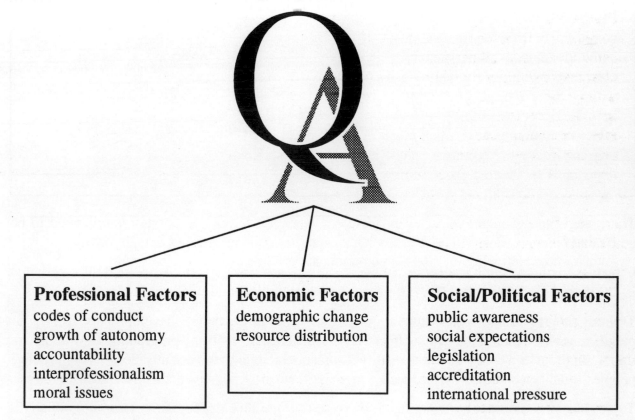

Professional Factors
codes of conduct
growth of autonomy
accountability
interprofessionalism
moral issues

Economic Factors
demographic change
resource distribution

Social/Political Factors
public awareness
social expectations
legislation
accreditation
international pressure

Each of these factors is now considered in turn.

❏ Professional Factors

● Codes of Conduct

Each profession has a Code of Conduct or a statement about professional behaviour which outlines professional rules. Boundaries are set for acceptable practice. If you, as a practitioner, operate outside your code of conduct, your licence to practise may be withdrawn. Quality assurance sets the Codes of Conduct into a broader framework. Professional bodies are also responsible for standards of training and qualification for practice.

● Growth of Autonomy and Accountability

In recent years professionals have taken increasing responsibility for their own practice. This has highlighted commitment to a consistent and accountable service–a major aim of a quality assurance system.

● Interprofessionalism

A quality service to clients often demands an interprofessional approach. This means that communication between the professions must be effective and efficient. Such communication is an integral part of quality assurance. Hence quality assurance has an important role to play in promoting and maintaining interprofessional relationships.

Let's have a look at communication in your workplace.

Activity

Name five persons at work with whom you regularly communicate;

✎ indicate their position within your organisation, and their professional background.

	name	position
1.		
2.		
3.		
4.		
5.		

Activity

Which of the following methods of communication do you use ?

✎ In each case, answer Yes or No.

Type of communication	answer
❏ meetings	
–formal	_____
–informal	_____
❏ ward rounds	_____
❏ written correspondence	
–formal	_____
–informal	_____
❏ telephone	_____
❏ other (please specify)	_____

34

Activity

For every method that you use, determine whether you consider this communication to be:

    –effective?

    –appropriate?

✎ Using the following table, answer Yes or No as appropriate. (Definitions of these two characteristics are given in the glossary, if you wish to check them).

Type of communication	effective	appropriate
❑ meetings		
–formal	_____	_____
–informal	_____	_____
❑ ward rounds	_____	_____
❑ written correspondence		
–formal	_____	_____
–informal	_____	_____
❑ telephone	_____	_____
❑ other (please specify)	_____	_____

Activity

Circle any 'no' responses in the above table.

✎ Jot down your main reasons for these negative responses.

You have identified an area that could form the basis of a quality improvement problem.

● **Moral Issues**

There is a moral obligation on everyone working in health care to provide a responsible and caring service to every client. Moral dilemmas can arise where a few people benefit from a very expensive care programme. The same expenditure in a low technology area could benefit many more clients. Further, the moral beliefs of individual health care professionals may affect the type of service they feel able to provide.

Quality assurance activities encourage open debate about the nature and extent of provision. They therefore help to ensure that moral judgements are only made after careful scrutiny of all the possible options.

❑ Economic Factors

• Demographic Change

Changing demography compels the adoption of quality assurance in health care. For example, existing population changes will lead to a society with an increasing number of dependent people whose health care must be paid for by the economically active. Therefore, there is a growing need for an efficient and economically run health care service. This is now becoming a sensitive political issue as choices are made and priorities established.

• Resource Distribution

The National Health Service is the largest employer in Britain. It is accountable for both the service it provides and the resources it uses. Quality assurance provides objective evidence for this accountability. It establishes that the service delivered is appropriate and meets clients' needs at an acceptable cost. It also supports individual accountability—as demanded by general management—and is an essential element in the evolution of service contracts. Finally, it provides a basis on which clients could choose between different suppliers of care.

❑ Social / Political Factors

• Public Awareness

Pressure from society is creating the need for a more efficient health service. The public generally are better informed about health care and their rights to health care. They are more inclined to use formal complaint procedures or the Ombudsman to achieve justice when a seemingly unacceptable level of service is received. More and more, the client's voice is being heard in respect of health care issues. In the past, clients have felt excluded from the professional decision-making process and were poorly informed about their treatment. A quality assurance system should ensure that the client's opinion is taken into account and that the client is consulted about treatment. Such consultation can even be regarded as the client's moral right.

• Social Expectations

Changing social expectations are another reason for quality assurance in health care. There is a growing number of consumer bodies which campaign for the rights of individuals or groups. Some of these have drawn up quality standards for use in client care settings. The National Association for the Welfare of Children in Hospital and The Association of Community Health Councils of England and Wales have published lists of what patients and relatives ought to expect of their Health Services. The media are often keen to take up such issues and to campaign for improved service.

• Legislation

The law clearly has a voice in maintaining standards in health care. Many minimal standards for practice are already agreed in law and form part of the quality assurance programmes of health care personnel. For example the Data Protection Act controls computerised information; the Medicines Act controls the use of drugs; the Nurses, Midwives and Health Visitors Act controls the education of these groups; and The Control of Substances Hazardous to Health Act limits the use of noxious substances. There are also strict laws covering the use of ionising radiation in radiography and radiotherapy departments.

The White Paper 'Working for Patients' (1989) and the resulting Health Service Reform Bill required health care professionals to confront quality assurance issues. To quote Nichol, 'The White Paper has emphasised the high importance which Ministers attach to quality of care and the provision of a service which is sensitive to the needs of its customers across the NHS.... In particular, we will be looking at how far health authorities are taking a forward-looking and systematic approach to quality of service and customer relations, and how far Regions and Districts can be confident that their quality statements are being translated into tangible benefits on the ground'.

● Accreditation

In Britain, private nursing homes need a licence to operate and are inspected by officers of the local Health Authority. In the USA, there is a statutory requirement for hospitals to be audited and accredited if they are to receive public funding. Accreditation of hospitals in Britain is being considered.

● International Pressure

The international political forum also has its effect on the health service. As a member of the World Health Organisation, Britain was committed to the development of quality assurance systems in health care by 1990. Several United Nations organisations also comment on health care standards.

In this section, you have seen that there are many reasons for the importance of quality assurance in health care. These include professional, economic, and social/political factors.

Activity

At the beginning of this section, you jotted down some of your own points. Would you make any changes to them now that you have worked through this section ?

✎ Add to your ideas if necessary.

Now that you know what quality assurance is and why it is needed in health care, it will be interesting to see how it evolved in the U.K.

3.3 How has quality assurance evolved in the U.K.?

Objectives:
By the end of this section you will be able to:
- trace the development of quality assurance in U.K. industry;
- trace the development of quality assurance in health care professions in the U.K.;
- identify how professional groups have responded to the evolution of quality assurance.

Quality and quality assurance are not new concepts, but their formalised adoption has been a slow process both in industry and in the service sectors.

Since industry has led the way, we shall begin by tracing the industrial development of a formal system of quality appraisal and action.

In the Middle Ages, merchant guilds were notable upholders of quality of goods produced by their members. For example, cloth bearing the Colchester guild mark was renowned for its high quality. In general during this period goods were handcrafted. This enabled self-inspection of work to ensure that high quality products reached the client. With the advent of technology allowing production of goods on a larger scale, self-inspection was no longer viable. Other methods of ensuring quality were required. This period saw the formation of professional organisations such as the Institution of Civil Engineers. Its aim was to promote and develop the knowledge and best practice of all categories of civil engineering. This led to the development and publication of British Standards that stipulated specifications for engineering materials.

The need for quality considerations was highlighted during World War I, when failure of British aircraft engines behind enemy lines resulted in the loss of trained pilots. From 1850 onwards, there had been a significant change in the scale and diversity of industry. Mass production evolved. This was a move away from the individual skilled craftsman to a team of less skilled operators who each performed one task in a sequence of line operations. That is, no one person had control or responsibility over the end product. This led to the development of inspection techniques. An inspector independently checked the quality of the finished product before it was dispatched to the client. Any unacceptable product was returned for reworking, or scrapped. The manufacturer thus incurred additional costs when substandard goods were produced.

The change in quality focus from inspection to the more efficient and cost-effective approach of structuring and managing a system for product quality took decades. During the 1930s and 1940s some companies developed and used statistical techniques to monitor the quality of produced goods. Throughout the 1950s and 1960s British manufacturers in general saw no reason to change either their production methods, which were geared to quantity not quality, or their management philosophy. It was during the recession of the 1970s that manufacturers recognised the need to change. Customers were becoming increasingly interested in quality and as a result trade was being lost to foreign imports. Thus the need for quality improvement across UK industry became of vital importance during the 1970s and 1980s in order to contain costs and compete with imports. Statistical techniques were used to improve quality and new techniques were developed specifically for this purpose. Slowly techniques such as Statistical Process Control, Quality Circles, Quality Assurance systems and philosophies such as Total Quality Management were implemented by industry.

Such strategies had played a significant role in quality improvement in Japanese industry post World War II. In the West, the first attempt to standardise quality had been in America in connection with defence contracts. These formed the basis for a series of three standards designed for NATO use and a series of three analogous specifications called Defence Standards used in the United Kingdom (1976). These latter standards were quality system specifications covering design, manufacture, inspection and test. They were the requirements to which firms wishing to bid for contracts from the Ministry of Defence had to conform. The NATO standards formed the basis of the first version of BS5750 (1979), which was a quality standard written for industry in general. Compliance with this standard was taken as objective evidence that a firm had specified a quality system and was working to it. The later version of this British standard was the basis of the international quality standard (ISO9000). The advent of an open European market in 1992 forced many manufacturers, large and small, to become accredited BS5750 holders.

Quality assurance has had a high profile in health care since the late 1980s. Many of the concepts and components in industrial quality assurance systems had parallels in the health care setting.

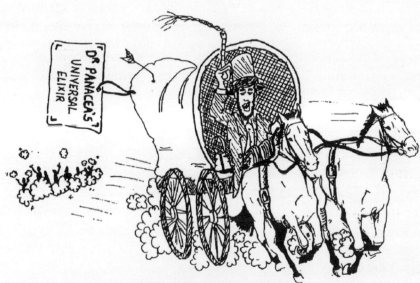
'Early Quality Assurance'

Concern for the quality of care is as old as medicine itself. Individual practitioners from Hippocrates to Florence Nightingale have recorded their observations of poor quality care and made recommendations for improvement. The first formal systems for the assurance of quality care, however, developed alongside the gradual professionalisation of medicine, nursing and other health professions. As early as the 16th century the Royal College of Physicians made reference in its founding charter to the need to 'uphold standards for public benefit'. In most cases the Colleges and other professional associations took their responsibility for 'upholding standards' to include regulation of education and training, control of admission, and development of powers of dismissal from the profession on grounds of malpractice. Until very recently, however, few provided anything beyond the broadest guidelines for the delivery of sound quality care by qualified members of the profession.

Since the establishment of the National Health Service in 1948 concern for the quality of care delivered has had a higher profile. Thus there has been a succession of inquiries and studies from the early 1950s onwards reporting on the incidence and circumstances of maternal death and perioperative death; on the use of Caesarean section; on cardiac and thoracic surgery; and on regional variations in access to care.

Formal standards and inspection and monitoring procedures have been developed for radiology, nuclear medicine and aspects of medical laboratory practice. The Royal College of General Practitioners launched a 'quality initiative' in 1985, and as early as 1965 the Royal College of Nursing set up its 'Standards of Care' project which has now developed into a major programme of research, development and education. Guidelines and standards have recently been produced by the professional bodies for physiotherapy, for occupational therapy, for dietetics, for theatre nurses and for pharmacy; and similar documents will shortly be produced for speech therapists, chiropodists, dentists and no doubt other groups.

This flurry of professional activity is mirrored in a series of government reports and documents which drew attention to the need for a service which provided high quality care within available resources —in other words value for the taxpayers' money. The 1989 'Working for Patients' Working Paper 6 confronted the issue directly and recommended the establishment of formal systems of 'medical audit' for both hospital and community care.

It is clear that both government and the professions have now recognised the importance of quality assurance in health care. There is considerable activity throughout the National Health Service and in private practice in discussing, piloting and setting up quality assurance procedures. All health professionals are going to be involved in some such system.

Activity
Go to your library or consult with senior colleagues and try to find out what your own professional organisation has published on 'quality assurance', 'medical/clinical audit', or 'professional standards'.

3.4 What does quality cost?

Objectives
By the end of this section you will be able to identify:
- costs of lack of quality;
- quality system costs.

Costs are an important factor in any business or organisation and health care is no exception. In general, costs are identified and recorded with respect to the performance of various functions, for example, specific categories of treatment, clerical assistance, building maintenance, laundry services. Quality related costs are often hidden or scattered among various accounts. It is important to identify and collate these costs to provide information on areas where quality improvements could be made.

Activity
It is worthwhile pausing here to query what is meant by the term 'costs' in the context of quality health care.

✎ Using a dictionary jot down its definitions of cost.

You have probably written words or phrases concerned with the monetary meaning of cost e.g. amount, price, charge; but note, too, its use to convey distress, suffering, sacrifice, pain. In a health care context these may characterise important costs to the client. A comparison of these and monetary costs is contentious and controversial. We shall not attempt this, but merely offer you a framework that will enable you to identify both monetary and non-monetary costs associated with quality.

It is useful to adopt the industrial distinction between costs incurred through a lack of quality or a 'poor' service, and costs incurred to provide and monitor a quality service (Juran, 1988; Feigenbaum, 1961):

- ❑ costs of lack of quality:
    - –failure costs,
    - –utilisation costs;
- ❑ quality system costs:
    - –appraisal costs,
    - –prevention costs.

❏ Failure costs

Failure costs are due to not doing the right thing in the right place at the right time. We need to add to this, in the right way and by the right personnel. This includes:

–not meeting agreed standards of care;

–setting standards inappropriate to client needs;

–setting standards that allow a client to receive incompatible treatments from different professionals;

–treating conditions that are capable of detection at an earlier stage of development when treatment costs and client costs would be lower;

–use of inappropriate materials, drugs and equipment necessitating the provision of further treatment and perhaps leading to a protracted period of care;

–miscommunication between people in the health care team leading to additional costs to rectify resultant incorrect actions and causing inconvenience to the client;

–incorrect treatment or incompetence during the provision of health care, possibly leading to liability costs.

❏ Utilisation costs

Utilisation costs are incurred when resources are not used efficiently and effectively. For example:

–inappropriate use of skills such that personnel are given tasks inconsistent with their ability, training and experience;

–under-utilisation of personnel and equipment that results in the potential quality of care not being reached;

–over-utilisation of materials and drugs resulting in excessive costs and waste;

–over-utilisation of personnel due to unnecessary appointments, unnecessary tests and treatment resulting in additional monetary costs and in additional waiting time for some clients;

–over-utilisation of equipment such that it is poorly maintained and infrequently calibrated.

Loss in morale and loss in goodwill are controversial quality costs that arise when practitioners' expectations of the system or organisation are not satisfied.

Activity

Refer back to the examples of utilisation costs.

✎ From your own working experience, jot down specific examples of instances when resources have not been used efficiently or effectively.

❑ Appraisal costs

Appraisal costs are incurred by administering a monitoring system that appraises and assesses the quality of care. Some appraisal techniques are discussed in unit two.

❑ Prevention costs

Prevention costs are incurred performing activities that are aimed at keeping failure and appraisal costs to a minimum. These activities include:

–development and maintenance of a quality system;
–development and improvement of standards;
–educating personnel about quality;
–providing continuing training of personnel.

Theoretically, the cost of implementing a quality assurance system should be outweighed by the resultant savings through improved efficiency, effectiveness and client satisfaction.

Finally in this unit we will guide you to sources of information about quality assurance.

3.5 How do you find out about quality assurance?

Objectives
By the end of 'How do you find out about quality assurance?' you will be able to:
- identify some methods of obtaining information both locally and nationally;
- identify key people and agencies who can provide you with information.

You may already know of some sources from whom you can obtain information about quality assurance.

Activity
Build up your own quality assurance information directory. Start by providing a source of information against each section in the directory below.

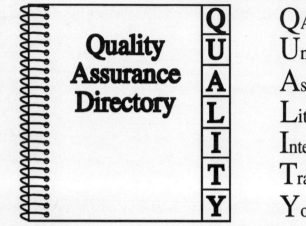

Quality Assurance Directory

QA manager in your district
Underlying directives
Associations interested in QA
Literature
Internal initiatives
Training
Your own professional body

You will find some sections easier to complete than others. Sources that you may have considered include:

Quality Assurance Manager

–District QA Manager; or, alternatively,
–District General Manager; or,
–Professional Manager.

Underlying Directives

–legislation past, present and awaited;
–resource management initiatives;
–contracting of service details.

Associations

–the British Standards Institution,
- an accreditation body for the national (and international) standard on quality assurance;
–the Department of Trade and Industry,
- provides some publications free on request;
–the Health Advisory Service;
–the Institute of Quality Assurance,
- concerned with the promotion of quality in manufacturing, production and service industries;

–The King's Fund Quality Assurance Centre,
- also provides a Quality Assurance Information Service;
- and an Information Exchange scheme;
–the World Health Organisation;
–the Royal College of Nursing Quality Assurance Network, (Q.U.A.N.),
- set up under the auspices of the Royal College of Nursing;
–your local university or polytechnic.

Literature

–U.K., European and world wide books, journals and articles;
–newspapers and magazines reflecting some of society's views and expectations;
–national reports publishing results of specific studies;
–Quality Assurance Abstracts, from DHSS;
–King's Fund Quality Assurance Centre bibliographic service;
–National Association of Quality Assurance in Health Care (which has regional groups).

Internal Initiatives

–peer group activity;
–activities of professional groups;
–district working parties;
–special interest groups.

Training

–by professional bodies,
- organised as uni- or interprofessional events at local and national level;
–by Health Authorities;
–by polytechnics and universities,
- short courses,
- undergraduate degree courses,
- postgraduate Masters courses.

Your Own Professional Body

–concerned with standard setting, definitions, working parties, directives, special interest groups, training days, working papers, directories.

Activity
Consider how you have found out about quality assurance. Do you feel that communication both locally and nationally is sufficient? If not, how might it be improved?

You may have suggested improvements such as regular circulars, an identified liaison person for each unit, or regular briefing sessions. You may also wish to consider how you could influence development of such improvements.

This completes the overview of Quality Assurance; you may wish to assess your understanding of the material by working through the following questions.

Self-assessment Question 5

✎ Complete the 'Summary of Quality Assurance' by inserting into the spaces provided the eight appropriate words from the list given below.

accountability	ensure	lack	objective	quality
appraisal	failure	managers	origins	subjective
continuing	important	monitor	professional	success
deliver	improvement	negligible	provision	unnecessary

Summary of Quality Assurance

Quality assurance is the responsibility of professionals and is the effective execution of all the actions concerned with attaining _____$_1$. It is aimed at improvement in the quality of care and at providing _____$_2$ evidence that a quality service is being delivered. The four basic steps in the quality assurance process are standard setting, appraising actual achievement, planning for _____$_3$ and taking action when required. These stages are performed repeatedly to give continuing improvement. A quality system enables a health care organisation to ensure that quality assurance activities take place, are documented and reported.

_____$_4$, economic and social factors underlie the need for quality assurance programmes in health care. Indeed, the economic recession of the 1970s was a prime force behind both industry and the service sector investigating and, albeit slowly, implementing quality assurance programmes. Although formalised quality assurance has its _____$_5$ in industry, its importation into health care did not necessitate a complete change in philosophy.

Costs are an _____$_6$ factor in health care, as in any business or organisation. Quality costs are usually segregated into costs incurred through a poor quality of service and costs incurred to provide and monitor a quality service. The former include _____$_7$ and utilisation costs, and the latter _____$_8$ and prevention costs.

Information on quality assurance is available from many sources, for example quality assurance managers, literature, various associations, training organisations and professional bodies.

Self-assessment Question 6

✎ Suggest a definition of quality assurance.

On a scale of 1 (low confidence) to 5 (high confidence) mark how confident you are about your definition:

scale   1   2   3   4   5

Return to your original definition of quality assurance (page 7). Are there any differences?

When you have completed this question turn to the glossary and compare your definition.

Self-assessment Question 7

Think carefully about the following statements.

Indicate whether you agree or disagree by ticking one of the columns.

✎ Jot down a reason for your choice.

Statement	Agree	Disagree	Reason
1. Quality assurance is unnecessary, since all health professionals work to a code of conduct.			
2. Quality care can be delivered only if the client is involved in decision making.			
3. A quality assurance programme aims to provide an efficient and effective service to the client.			

Self-assessment Question 8

✎ For each statement, decide whether it is true or false. Circle your answer.

1) Under-utilisation costs are incurred when excessive material is used or unnecessary appointments are made.

    True/False

2) Prevention costs are incurred by developing systems aimed at the elimination of unacceptable goods or services.

    True/False

3) Quality Assurance is a continual process aimed at improving services delivered to clients.

    True/False

4) Quality Assurance is solely the business of the quality manager.

    True/False

Self-assessment Question 9

✎ Jot down four sources of information about quality assurance:

1.

2.

3.

4.

Solutions to self-assessment questions

Solution to Self-assessment Question 5

space	word
1	quality
2	objective
3	improvement
4	professional
5	origins
6	important
7	failure
8	appraisal

Solution to Self-assessment Question 6

As with quality, it is not easy to frame a definition of quality assurance in one sentence. Now that you have worked through unit one, you are probably more confident about your understanding of quality assurance. This will increase as you work through unit two.

Solution to Self-assessment Question 7

1. We disagree with this statement.

Quality assurance is **necessary** even though health professionals work to a code of conduct.

Several incentives for adopting quality assurance in health care were given in section 3.2. An important point to stress is that quality assurance provides objective evidence of the satisfaction of specified client requirements. This is central to the concept of purchaser-provider contracts.

2. If we have convinced you that quality assurance is concerned with satisfying the client's requirements, then your response will say that it is important that the client is involved in some way in the decision making process. That is not to say that the client dictates what treatment they need. You will meet some ways in which to involve clients in unit two of this workbook.

3. All the material presented in unit one supports the statement that a quality assurance programme aims to provide an efficient and effective service to clients (at an acceptable cost).

Solution to Self-assessment Question 8

1) False.

Over-utilisation costs are incurred when excessive material is used or unnecessary appointments are made.

2) True.

Prevention costs are incurred by developing systems aimed at the elimination of unacceptable goods or services.

It is important to remember that costs (monetary and non-monetary) will be incurred when setting up quality assurance systems. Attention to resources is therefore essential. The costs of not having such a system must also be considered.

3) True.

Quality assurance is a continual process aimed at improving services delivered to clients. More detail is given on this in unit two.

4) False.

Quality assurance is everyone's business. A quality service cannot be achieved unless everyone is committed to quality improvement.

Solution to Self-assessment Question 9

You may wish to compare your sources with those provided in section 3.5.

ASSESSING AND IMPROVING QUALITY

52

4 Introduction to Assessing and Improving Quality

In unit one you met concepts underlying quality and quality assurance. From this work you will have appreciated that quality is a dynamic concept and not a static one; that quality is everyone's business; and that judging quality requires agreement of standards. You also learned about the industrial origins of quality assurance and traced its development in health care.

In unit two, you will explore how you might take part in quality assurance within your own professional practice.

4.1 The quality system

Objective
By the end of this section you will be able to:
- describe the 'quality climate' in your own area of professional practice.

In earlier sections (particularly 2.4 and 3.1) we stressed the importance of involving everyone in quality improvement. We also suggested that it was vitally important to secure a genuine commitment to quality improvement from senior managers and policy makers. Ideally, such commitment and universal involvement is expressed by top management in a quality policy which is realised through the implementation and maintenance of a quality system. This quality system could follow the requirements laid down in the British Standard, BS 5750, which has been used by industry for some time and is now being adapted for introduction into the service sector.

A recent survey of quality management in the NHS (Dalley and Carr-Hill, 1991) found that the majority of District Health Authorities in England and Wales had made a formal commitment to quality assurance. These Authorities had begun to designate responsibility for quality assurance to named senior staff. They varied considerably, however, in the pattern and aims of their quality activities; in the way that professionals and middle managers were involved; and in the effectiveness of communication about quality.

Activity

✎ Look back to section 3.1 where we introduced the following list of important features in a quality system. Rate your own area of professional practice by giving a score out of 10 for each of these features. (A score of 1 indicates absence of the feature; a score of 10 indicates presence of the feature with no improvement being possible).

FEATURE	SCORE
commitment from top management	_____
commitment from all personnel	_____
clear responsibilities for quality activities	_____
willingness to change	_____
accurate documentation	_____
effective communication at all levels of the organisation	_____
ongoing training programme on quality	_____
ongoing skills training programme	_____

Now decide to what extent you feel you work in a 'quality climate'.

In health care, quality assurance often begins with practitioners who are close to the day to day process of care. The success or failure of a quality initiative will obviously be influenced by the quality system or quality culture within which it takes place. On the other hand, a successful quality initiative might help to change a previously unsupportive organisational setting.

Some Health Authorities and many service industries have addressed the issue of quality culture by the introduction of a Total Quality Management programme. These programmes are based upon the belief that quality is what the customer says it is and that a belief in quality must be thoroughly integrated into the organisation. Fundamental to such programmes is identification of both internal and external customers and clear clarification of their needs.

In the rest of this unit, we discuss relatively small scale quality assurance initiatives which can be undertaken by groups of professionals at any organisational level. We assume a moderately supportive organisational setting but make no assumptions about the particular system of quality management.

4.2 The quality wheel

Objective:
By the end of this section you will be able to:
- use a quality wheel to show the stages in the quality assurance process.

In section 3.1, quality assurance was defined as being concerned with all activities involved in attaining quality. The basic stages in quality assurance were shown in a simple wheel.

Activity

✎ Complete the framework of the quality wheel shown below.

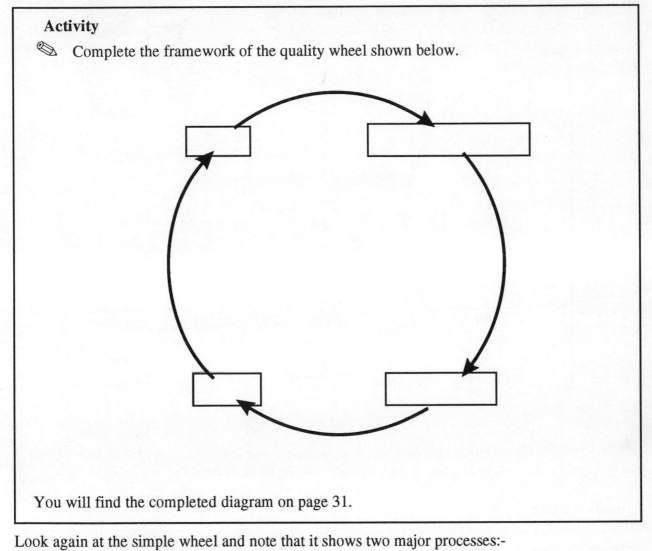

You will find the completed diagram on page 31.

Look again at the simple wheel and note that it shows two major processes:-
  ❑ **quality appraisal**
    –setting standards,
    –appraising actual achievement;
  ❑ **quality action**
    –planning for improvement,
    –taking action when necessary.

The basic steps in quality appraisal and quality action are revised in this unit to guide you through the stages in a quality assurance initiative. The amended wheel (which has been adapted from Lang, 1984) is shown in diagrams 8 and 9 and an overview of these stages follows.

❑ **quality appraisal**

A quality group is established which sets standards, selects appropriate measurement techniques to evaluate what is happening in practice, and then compares observed practice with the agreed standards.

During early discussions, the group identifies a focus for the quality assurance initiative and clarifies beliefs and values about practice. This is important. For example, some professionals may believe that old people have poor recovery ability. Other professionals may believe that, with active rehabilitation, older people can return to active participation in the community. People holding these contrasting views would set different standards.

Diagram 8.   Quality Appraisal

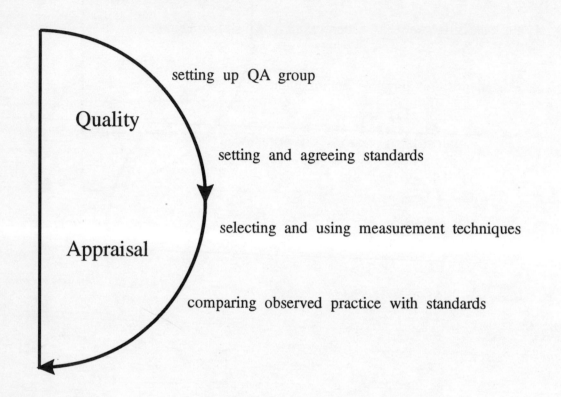

Quality

Appraisal

setting up QA group

setting and agreeing standards

selecting and using measurement techniques

comparing observed practice with standards

Whilst setting standards and measuring their achievement is interesting, it is of little benefit unless the acquired information is used. Using the information is quality action.

❑ **quality action**

When observed practice is compared with agreed standards, differences may become apparent. Any differences are investigated and action plans are discussed. Inevitably resources will affect decisions taken at this stage. For example, an old building with poor facilities cannot be replaced overnight, but conditions within that building can be improved—often with little expenditure.

Several options for improvement are identified, the quality assurance group selects the most suitable plan, implements it, and finally reappraises the situation to check that the planned improvements have actually occurred.

Diagram 9   Quality Action

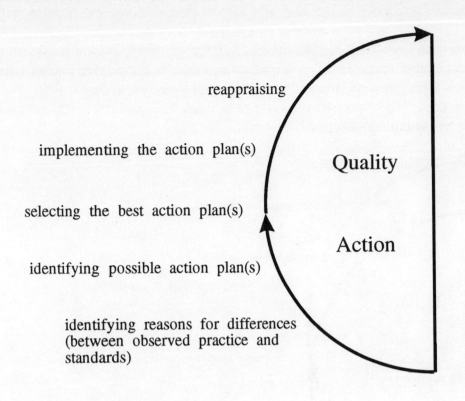

reappraising

implementing the action plan(s)

selecting the best action plan(s)

identifying possible action plan(s)

identifying reasons for differences
(between observed practice and
standards)

Quality

Action

We will now examine in greater detail each of the stages in quality appraisal.

57

5 The Steps in Quality Appraisal

To achieve this objective we will work through the stages shown in diagram 10.

Diagram 10   Quality Appraisal

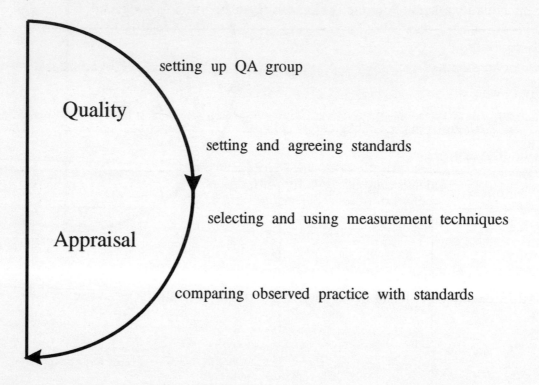

5.1 Setting up a quality assurance group

A quality assurance group is a team of people who meet together to undertake quality assurance activities. Working in a group has advantages and disadvantages. Its advantages lie in bringing different viewpoints together. Its disadvantages are associated with getting people to work together effectively.

The following points will be discussed in this section:
❑ group size
❑ group membership
❑ group effectiveness
❑ organisation of meetings

❑ **Group size**
Group size depends to some extent on the scope of the intended quality assurance initiative. A group with overall responsibility for quality assurance throughout a unit might be large and therefore need to set up subgroups to tackle specific issues.

On the other hand, a group considering quality issues in the service delivered by one specific ambulance crew, might involve only two or three people.

There is some evidence to suggest that eight is a good size for a group where the main task is discussion and problem solving. This size allows full contribution from individual members.

The rest of this section is based on a quality assurance group with a relatively specific area of responsibility and between four and ten members.

❑ Group membership

Setting up a quality assurance group is like setting up any other work group.

Activity
Consider an aspect of your own work in which quality assurance might be useful.
✎ Jot down a list of six or seven people you would like to include in a group set up to consider this aspect. Identify the position of each individual and say why you would include them.

Aspect of Work

Name	Position	Reason for Inclusion

Consider your list. You may have included some people primarily for their position, but others for their special knowledge and skills. Some may have been included because they are easy to work with.

Check your list again.
Have you included a client–or a member of a client pressure group?
Have you included all of the people your quality assurance activity might directly affect?
Have you included someone who has access to negotiation for resources?

❑ Group effectiveness

You will have experience of different groups—project groups, medical teams, or groups of friends. Inevitably some will have been more successful than others.

Activity

Recall a group of which you have been a member which was successful in achieving its goals and one which was largely unsuccessful.

✎ Jot down some of the features of the effective group and of the ineffective group.

Features of Effective Group	Features of Ineffective Group

Your experience may or may not be typical, but compare the features that you thought important with those set out by the social psychologist Michael Argyle (1969). He suggests that effective groups have the following characteristics. They:

- meet frequently;
- meet informally as well as formally;
- make jokes and mention personal matters even when they are working;
- have similar attitudes and values;
- agree upon the purpose of the group;
- have developed an implicit (and sometimes explicit) agreement about division of labour and distribution of relevant tasks and roles;
- have sound discussion skills;
- include someone who is particularly good at leading discussion.

Few quality assurance groups will take up this ideal form instantaneously. It is more likely that effectiveness will begin to emerge after the first two or three meetings. The initiator of the group might help by talking to each participant individually to establish agreement on the purpose of the group and to allay any potential fears or anxieties.

The leader of the group may need to brush up on chairmanship skills:

Are they good at summarising other people's contributions?
Do they ask contributors to clarify their comments?
Do they look at other members encouragingly while they speak?
Are they good at staying quiet while others contribute?

Another feature that you may have considered in the last activity is whether group members were volunteers. One school of thought suggests that quality assurance groups should be made up entirely of volunteers. However this approach may mean that people who did not volunteer are unaware of developments within the group and therefore are unable to understand or support change. A different approach suggests that quality assurance groups should be 'natural workgroups' so that everyone is involved whether they are enthusiasts for change or natural conservatives. A disadvantage with this approach is that the workgroup may not have representatives from senior levels who can help to authorise change.

❑ **Organisation of meetings**

Activity
Recall a successful discussion, problem–solving or committee group of which you have been a member.

✎ Jot down the organisational features that helped it to be an effective group.

You may have included some of the following:
- meetings lasted less than $1^1/2$ hours;
- a clear agenda was prepared;
- the frequency of meetings was agreed;
- members were informed of the time and venue and plenty of notice was given;
- meetings were held away from the immediate workplace so as to be free from interruption;
- good records were kept of
    - participants at each meeting,
    - decisions made,
    - action to be taken (by whom and by when);
- records were sent to non-group members whose support might be required at a later stage in the initiative.

All of these features help to ensure the smooth and effective operation of a quality assurance group. In addition, some health authorities and professional groups have set up teams of facilitators who have experience in helping groups to initiate and carry out quality assurance. They are particularly skilled in helping groups to run smoothly and effectively.

In this section you have considered some aspects of setting up a quality assurance group. Now let's consider the first stage in the group's activities.

5.2 Setting and agreeing standards

> **Objectives**
> By the end of this section you will be able to:
> - identify a suitable topic for standard setting;
> - write a standard;
> - write criteria which relate to that standard.

You met standards and criteria in section 2.3 and discussed who should be involved in setting standards in section 2.4. Since standard setting is a key element in any quality assurance initiative, it is studied in more detail in this section.

The steps used here in writing standards are derived from the work done by Lang (1984), Schroeder et al (1986), Kitson and Kendall (1986) and expanded upon in the Royal College of Nursing system DySSSy (1990). There are many different methods of writing standards. We have chosen to follow this approach because of its clarity and its increasing popularity in nursing and other professions. It is in use in the United Kingdom, Republic of Ireland, Holland, Scandinavia, Iceland and Israel. The basic steps involve discussion and agreement on:
- ❑ topic
- ❑ subtopics
- ❑ care group
- ❑ standard statement
- ❑ criteria

❑ Topic

A topic is an area of activity or aspect of care for which a quality assurance group wishes to write a standard. When a topic is selected, there is usually a general set of clients under consideration. Specific membership will be defined as the quality assurance group progresses through setting a standard.

❑ Subtopics

A subtopic is a smaller more specific area of the topic which has been singled out for particular attention.

Most quality groups begin by setting topics which are quite broad and subtopics can be identified in most cases. For example, if the topic selected was maintaining a safe environment, subtopics could be the prevention of patient falls, education for staff or relatives on safety, or prevention of accidents with particular pieces of equipment. Thus, a range of smaller, more precise subtopics may be identified from one broad topic.

Standards are written on the subtopics, therefore it is important to define them clearly and precisely. They must be understood and agreed upon by all members of the group. Time spent on ensuring this is time well spent.

Activity

✎ Get together with at least two colleagues and decide upon a topic for standard setting.

Topic:

Individually write lists of three distinct subtopics.

      1.

      2.

      3.

Now, as a group agree and jot down a list of three subtopics. These subtopics will be used in later activities.

      Subtopic 1:

      Subtopic 2:

      Subtopic 3:

Here are some questions that a quality assurance group needs to consider when deciding on topics and subtopics:

- Is the selected topic/subtopic within the group's area of responsibility?
- Will professional colleagues outside the group agree with selection of this topic/subtopic?
- Will management agree with selection of this topic/subtopic?
- With reasonable time and effort, will concentration on this topic/subtopic lead to an improvement in the quality of care?

If the answer to any of these questions is NO and is likely to remain so another topic should be selected.

Activity

Return to the three subtopics that you chose in the last activity and check them against these questions. If necessary, revise your choice.

❑ Care group

The care group is the set of clients for whose care the standard is to be written. It could be all patients on a particular unit, or all babies under 2 months in the community, or all new admissions. The standards written should relate to the whole group and be seen as relevant to each member. In some settings individual intervention strategies may be written to supplement standards for the more global care group.

❑ Standard statement

The standard statement is the hub on which the other elements of the standard revolve. It is an agreed level of performance appropriate to the care group and relevant to the selected subtopic. It specifies a desirable, acceptable and achievable level of care.

A standard statement should:

- be clearly written;
- address an agreed subtopic;
- pertain to an agreed care group;
- be acceptable to relevant colleagues.

As you probably realised, the example standard statement is not totally precise and could therefore be difficult to measure. We now come to a crucial part of formulating standards – namely writing measurable criteria.

❑ **Criteria**

Criteria specify clearly and precisely the levels of performance which have to be achieved to satisfy the standard.

Your criteria may have stated how much choice the patients should have–for each course, from a list of what length–and so on. You probably found that it was more difficult to write criteria that depended on what you meant by 'nutritious' or on what it meant to be 'in line with the treatment schedule'. These are issues that a quality assurance group needs to discuss and clarify when writing criteria.

In section 2.3. we referred to Donabedian's work on quality assurance standards. He suggests that standards and criteria can be classified as one of three types:

- structure
- process
- outcome

● Structure criteria

These specify the level of resource provision needed for achievement of a standard. They may refer to personnel, equipment, supplies, buildings, record systems, or (more fundamentally) finance. For our nutrition example, structure criteria include availability of a variety of foodstuffs, competent kitchen staff and time to consult patients on their choices. An example structure criterion is: 'A dietitian is available on 24-hour call'.

● Process criteria

These specify the activities which must be undertaken to achieve a standard. They are the 'doing' part of the standard. They state who does what, to whom, when and how–when the standard is being achieved. For our nutrition example, some process criteria are:

–a dietitian assesses the patient's dietary restrictions on admission;
–a nurse ensures that menus are distributed to all patients each day.

● Outcome criteria

These specify the end results of care. As indicated in earlier sections, outcome criteria are the most important.

Commonly used outcome criteria involve :

–client satisfaction;
–client knowledge;
–client compliance;
–client function;
–recovery indicators.

Returning to our nutrition example, a possible outcome criterion is 'the patient is satisfied with the choice of food offered' or 'the client can state two reasons why they must adhere to their special diet'.

Activity
Which of the two outcome criteria is easier to use and why?

We think that the second one is easier to use. It is more precise and more easily agreed upon. The first criterion is less precise–how do you know when the client is 'satisfied'?

A typical proforma for writing standards is shown in Diagram 11 (Kitson and Kendall, 1986).

Diagram 11   Proforma for Standard Writing

Topic: Subtopic: Care Group: Standard Statement:				Appraisal date: Review date: Authorised by:	
No.	**Structure**	**No.**	**Process**	**No.**	**Outcome**

For any given standard on any given subtopic or topic, it is possible to write a great many criteria. Quality assurance groups, therefore, have to choose criteria which are both the best indicators of the achievement of standards and the easiest to use. One way to check criteria is to apply the 'AMOUR' principle. That is, are the criteria

Achievable?

Measurable?

Observable?

Understandable?

Reasonable?

● Achievable

We all practise within restraints of time and resources. Often, there is a difference between what is desirable and what can reasonably be expected in the circumstances.

When a quality group writes standard statements and criteria, it must choose between idealism and realism. If a realistic standard is set, members of a group can identify progress and congratulate themselves. From this point, they are likely to move forward in the continual quest for quality improvement and not become disillusioned by unattainable standards.

● Measurable

Measurability is the most important feature. A standard statement might not be worded in measurable terms but a criterion must be. When writing a criterion it is helpful to consider:-
- –How can a check be made that a criterion is being achieved?
- –How can the observed level of performance be evaluated?
- –How will people know whether it has been met?

A useful rule of thumb is–if it isn't measurable in some way don't include it as a criterion.

● Observable

For a phenomenon to be observable it must be detectable through the senses. If a criterion refers to unobservable phenomena it is impossible to determine whether or not it has been achieved. A criterion which uses vague terms such as 'appropriate empathy' is very difficult to use. It would be better to discuss what is understood by 'appropriate empathy' and to set an apparently crude criterion such as 'the therapist should look at the client when the client talks' or 'each client should have a daily opportunity to talk to the therapist'.

● Understandable

A criterion must be clearly understood by everyone who uses it. Vague terminology should be avoided and the quality assurance group should decide what is meant by 'appropriate' staffing levels or 'suitable' menu choices. The rule is always to be clear, objective and specific.

● Reasonable

To ensure quality is viewed as everyone's responsibility, it is important that those professionals not directly involved in the standard setting group do 'own' the standards. Therefore, colleagues, senior management and clients who have not been involved in formulating the standard and related criteria must be consulted for their comments. Colleagues whose professional practice is to be appraised must agree on their validity and acceptability. In other words, criteria must appear to be reasonable to all relevant colleagues.

Here is an example standard:

	**Topic:** Safety **Subtopic:** Prevention of harm in the event of a fire **Care Group:** All mobile patients on a 30 bedded surgical ward	**Appraisal date:** 30.1.91 **Review date:** 30.2.91 **Authorised by:**

Standard Statement: That all mobile patients on the ward understand, and are aware of, the hospital fire policy, and can evacuate the premises in the event of a fire, thus avoiding danger.

No.	Structure	No.	Process	No.	Outcome
1)	Stock of 30 fire information leaflets.	1)	Staff nurse gives a fire information leaflet to each patient on admission.	1)	Patient is in possession of a fire information leaflet.
2)	1 map identifying emergency escape routes.	2)	Staff nurse explains fire information leaflet to the patient.	2)	Patient understands the fire procedure.
3)	4 fire exits	3)	Staff nurse orientates patient to whereabouts of safety equipment on ward.	3)	Patient knows the position of the fire safety equipment on the ward.
4)	8 fire doors	4)	Staff nurse orientates patient to recognised safety zone.	4)	Patient can find the way to safety region.
5)	2 fire hoses	5)	Nurse ensures all O_2 points are clearly marked with No Smoking sign.	5)	If the patient is a smoker, the restricted smoking area is used whenever the patient smokes.
6)	4 fire extinguishers	6)	Staff nurse orientates patient to No Smoking zone.		
7)	2 fire blankets				
8)	2 fire alarms				
9)	1 fire policy				
10)	1 safety zone				
11)	1 smoking zone				
12)	15 No Smoking signs for each oxygen (O_2) point.				
13)	All staff have knowledge regarding fire policy.				

As you have seen, setting and agreeing standards is a complex process. This is summarised in Diagram 12.

Diagram 12.   The Elements of Standard Writing

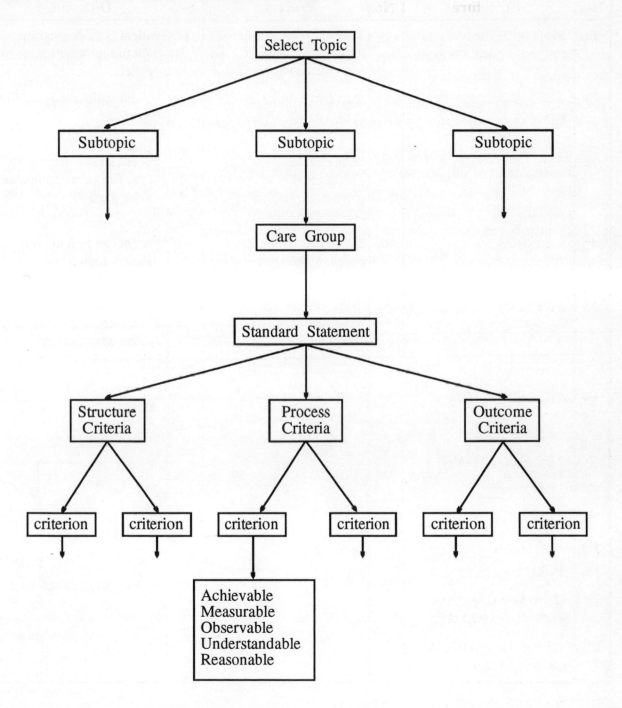

Once standards and criteria have been written, the next step in appraising quality of care is selecting and using measurement techniques to determine the extent to which standards have been met.

5.3 Selecting and using measurement techniques

Objectives
By the end of this section you will be able to :
- describe some techniques for measuring criteria;
- list some advantages and disadvantages of these techniques;
- identify some quality assurance measuring systems.

When setting standards and establishing criteria, it is important to consider when and how they will be monitored. The criteria which we have used so far have been relatively simple. Straightforward observation will reveal whether there are two fire hoses, one fire hose or none at all. All that is needed is a checklist. Other criteria may be far more complex and will require more sophisticated measurement techniques.

Standards can be appraised during or after the delivery of care. These techniques are referred to as concurrent and retrospective appraisal, respectively (Mayers et al, 1977).

Retrospective appraisal usually includes some combination of the following:
- ❑ **assessment** of clients' notes and other records (sometimes called **audit**);
- ❑ **interviews** with clients and perhaps with their relatives or friends, or with staff members;
- ❑ **questionnaires** administered to clients or their relatives or friends, or staff members;
- ❑ **conferences** held by relevant staff, clients etc.

Concurrent appraisal includes all of the above with the addition of:
- ❑ **direct observation** of care.

Diagram 13.   Types of Appraisal

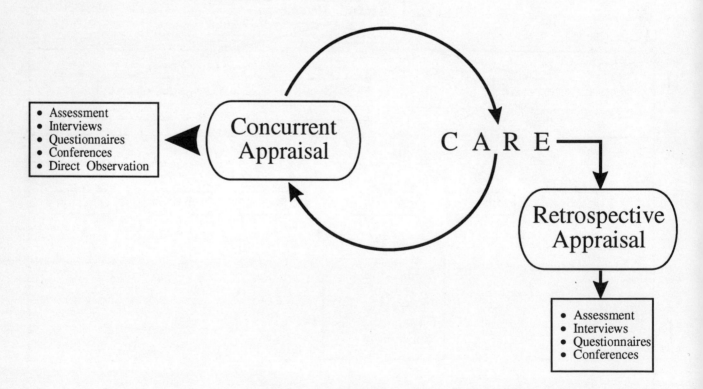

We now consider each of these measurement techniques.

❏ Assessment/audit

Assessment of clients' notes and other records is useful at the beginning of a quality assurance initiative. Information is readily available and easy for a quality assurance group to agree about.

Since this appraisal is based on records, however, it is only as good as the records themselves. If they are poor or incomplete, then the assessment of care quality will be inaccurate. On the other hand, people involved in keeping records can get very good at doing just that. Sometimes, perfect records are produced which bear little relationship to the standard of care provided. Care may even deteriorate because too much time is needed for the completion of the records. It is, therefore, very important that assessment is based on simple recording techniques which are easy to use and seem relevant to staff using them. A range of record based measurement systems have emerged, for example, Problem Oriented Medical Records (POMR) (Weed, 1971). This system, developed in the USA, is now widely used by occupational therapists and physiotherapists in the UK. It is designed to be used at a departmental level to determine the nature and quality of care offered to clients. It is commonly integrated into a clinical audit framework. Although it is primarily a means of evaluating the standards of a department as a whole, individual therapists commonly view this system as a means of monitoring the standards of their own individual intervention. In a similar way, nurses use care plans to monitor the quality of individual client care.

In summary, advantages and disadvantages of assessment/audit include:

advantages
- records are usually readily available;
- establishment of record based audit encourages good record keeping.

disadvantages
- assessment based on poor records will be inaccurate;
- excessive time spent on record keeping decreases time available for care.

❏ Interviews

Activity
✎ Jot down advantages and disadvantages you have experienced or anticipate from interviews with clients in relation to quality measurement.

advantages	disadvantages

Depending on the criteria being assessed, interviews may be structured or unstructured. Structured interviews have preset questions and possible answers. Returning to the nutrition example, a few structured questions may be all that is needed. For example:

'Did you get a chance to choose what you wanted to eat?
Please answer yes or no.'

and

'How many choices were there?
Please give a number.'

If these questions are repeated for each main meal, then the agreed criteria for the standard have been assessed. In such a structured situation, the role of the interviewer is largely to reassure the interviewee and to make sure they understand the questions and answer them clearly.

The interviewer has a larger role to play when interviews are unstructured or a mix of structured and unstructured. In an unstructured interview the interviewer has a clear idea of what they want to know, but leaves more room for the interviewee to put responses in context.
In the nutrition example, questions could begin with

'Did you enjoy your meals?'.

It would be up to the interviewer to use subsequent probing comments such as

'Really—why was that?'

or,

'I see—tell me more'.

This would uncover the importance and reality of choice for that particular individual. The structured interview might never discover that choices were exclusively between the dull and the disgusting, but even a semi-structured interview with a final question

'Is there anything else you would like to say about the food?'

would reveal such a state of affairs.

If the criteria being assessed are relevant to a large care group, a series of decisions must be made about who is to be interviewed. Any source of consistent bias must be avoided, for example, only interviewing male clients or clients cared for by a particular member of staff.

Interviewers who are known to clients may be able to get them to talk freely and to give specific and relevant detail. Their major disadvantage is that clients who have negative opinions may hold back for fear of giving offence. Many quality assurance initiatives have been criticised for assessing clients' satisfaction with care provided while they are still receiving care—in that context an interview can seem like blackmail!

In summary, advantages and disadvantages of interviews include:
advantages
- interviews can make sure that questions are understood and answers clearly given;
- interviews can make sure that the right clients provide the information;
- clients feel personally involved in their own care;
- clients have an opportunity to raise issues that may have been missed in designing the interview;
- in unstructured interviews, the interviewer can explore in depth the clients' attitudes and opinions, and can respond to clients' non-verbal cues.

disadvantages
- clients may find it difficult to give negative opinions;
- interviews are time consuming and, therefore, costly;
- the interviewer may unconsciously influence the answers given by the client.

❑ Questionnaires

Questionnaires, like interviews, can be structured or unstructured, in other words questions can be closed or open-ended.

Administration of questionnaires is a commonly used technique in quality assurance in health care. Unfortunately they are not always appropriate to the situation or client group. In addition many include misleading, biased questions. To help overcome such problems 'piloting' of any questionnaire is recommended before widespread use and interpretation.

The advantages and disadvantages of questionnaire use are widely documented and include the following:

advantages
- can be administered easily to a group from a wide geographical area;
- economical of time and money;
- each recipient is asked the same questions;
- interviewer bias is eliminated;
- if anonymous in nature, the respondent may be more prepared to be honest in the replies.

disadvantages
- if questions are unclear, inaccurate responses may be given;
- the style of the questionnaire, or wording of individual questions may direct the clients' responses;
- response rate is commonly low;
- they may not be completed by the intended client but by an informed carer with a differing view.

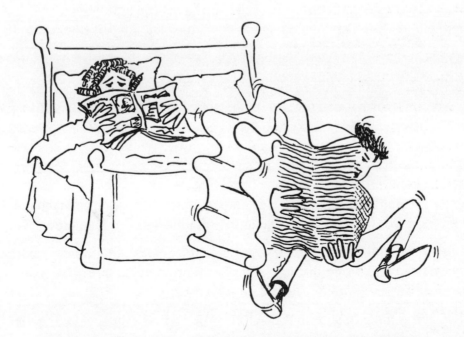

'They've sent us one of these short questionnaires again'

❑ Conferences

Conferences and discussions held by the interprofessional care team (possibly involving clients, relatives etc.) can yield useful information on the achievement of criteria. Their emphasis on quality distinguishes them from typical case conferences.

Their advantages and disadvantages include:

advantages
- involvement of all relevant individuals;
- flexibility in examining all aspects of a criterion rather than just those determined by a structured questionnaire or interview.

disadvantages
- the length of time they take;
- the inconvenience of assembling all of the relevant individuals;
- difficulty in interpreting the results of the discussion;
- bias resulting from personal relationships and status differences within the group;
- bias resulting from lack of objectivity about practice.

❏ Direct observation

Direct observation avoids some of the difficulties associated with reconstructing events from retrospective inspection of records, or from responses to interviewers or questionnaires. It may also be the only way to 'catch' the detail of care.

Who the observers are is important. Direct observation of some highly technical aspects of care is almost impossible for someone without sufficient specialist knowledge. On the other hand, a regular participant in a specialist group of care professionals may miss, or even distort, significant events. This is because they think they know what they are going to see and, therefore, forget to look!

The observer must:-
- be acceptable to those to be observed;
- be as unobtrusive as possible;
- have sufficient background to understand what is going on;
- be able to maintain some degree of objectivity.

Some quality assurance systems solve the problem by having groups of similar wards undergoing observation during the same period. Staff from each ward are then involved as observers of the other wards. When results are pooled, staff from each ward have been both observed and observer. Thus, they are better able to share experiences and to come to something like an accurate record.

Activity

Next time you go to coffee, make an agreement with one of your colleagues that you will both keep a record of what you observe in the coffee area during the first five minutes.

When you have completed your records, compare notes with your colleague. Discuss any differences in your observations and any difficulties you encountered.

You probably faced some problems in this activity. In the first instance, your colleagues may have decided they would rather not be observed. Even if they agreed, their behaviour may have been subtly (or not so subtly!) artificial. This is the first difficulty with direct observation. The behaviour of observed people is changed if they are aware of being the subject of attention. In the quality assurance context, colleagues being observed will be tempted to be 'on their best behaviour'.

A further difficulty encountered in direct observation is the problem of deciding what and when to record. As notes are made about one event, another one is unfolding and records are probably incomplete. Some of this difficulty is resolved if criteria are carefully specified, so that the observer has specific events to monitor. If the criteria are precise, they can be rephrased into questions which can be answered by 'yes', 'no' or 'not applicable'. It is also useful if criteria contain some notion of how often observations are to be made.

Checklists are an easy way to systematise observation during the process of care.
The advantages and disadvantages of direct observation thus include:

advantages
- immediacy;
- lack of retrospective bias.

disadvantages
- introduction of artificiality;
- observer bias due to ignorance;
- observer bias due to overinvolvement;
- the need to decide how often observations are to be recorded;
- inaccuracy of recording.

❑ Sampling
All techniques require some element of sampling:-
How many clients are to be interviewed?
How many colleagues are to be observed?
How many records are to be assessed?
In other words,
   What sample of the care group and their carers is to be selected for scrutiny?

These issues of sampling are discussed in detail in some of the referenced texts, but there are two main rules.
First,
   the sample selected must be unbiased—it must be as like the whole group as it can be.
Secondly,
   the sample must yield measurements in a quantity which the group can realistically handle—there is no point in administering a large number of lengthy questionnaires if it will take 18 months to analyse the answers.

These two rules of sampling are at odds with each other. The representativeness rule might suggest a large sample (or even 100% inclusion); but the practicality rule a small one. The quality assurance group decides on the balance. The group might consult someone who is experienced in this area.

❑ Systems for appraising standards
One way to ease the problems of measurement is to use a measurement technique which someone else has devised and used successfully in a context similar to your own.

As quality assurance in health care has developed, a number of 'off the shelf' techniques for the concurrent appraisal of quality has become available. A few of them are mentioned here.

One very popular technique is the Monitor system. This has been used as an index of quality in nursing and began as an Anglicised version of the American Rush-Medicus System. Monitor deals with process criteria, concentrating to a large degree on the stages of the Nursing Process.

Several other appraisal techniques have been developed for nursing including Wandelt and Ager's 'QUALPACS' (1974) and Daugherty and Mason's 'EXCELCARE' (Price Waterhouse, 1987). Occupational therapy, physiotherapy and speech therapy professions are not making use of 'off the shelf' systems, but are working within a framework of nationally produced standards. These and standards produced by special interest groups are made more specific at a local and client level. Use of standards in this manner has led to growing use of POMR and similar record-based systems as a means of monitoring quality standards in all areas of clinical intervention. In the USA and Australia, systems similar to POMR have been used for accreditation purposes.

With all such quality appraisal techniques, it is important to weigh convenience against appropriateness. It is convenient to select an 'off the shelf' technique, but will it measure the criteria the quality group wish to appraise, or will it measure some other factors decided upon by its inventor? 'Off the shelf' techniques are not 'custom made' to suit a specific area of practice. They are very good at producing an overall indicator of the quality of care for a particular care setting, but they are not easily adaptable to the measurement of specific standards written by a quality group. If they are modified to meet the needs of a specific setting or care group, then measures produced are no longer comparable with those of other similar groups using the 'off the shelf' technique.

An obvious criticism of 'off the shelf' techniques is that they have not been developed by the group which is going to use them. Arguably, therefore, the group may not be as knowledgeable or as enthusiastic about them as it could be. Further discussion and comparison of 'off the shelf' techniques are given in the texts to which we refer at the end of this workbook.

Activity

✎ Jot down any techniques that are being used in your work setting.

In this section we have considered ways of tackling the measurement of criteria. It is apparent that quality assurance groups must bear issues of measurement in mind throughout the process of determining topics, subtopics, standards and criteria.

The next step in the cycle of quality appraisal is comparing the measurements obtained with the standards and criteria set.

5.4 Comparing observed practice with standards

Objectives
By the end of this section you will be able to:
- decide when practice should be compared with standards;
- decide who should carry out the comparison;
- describe potential difficulties in comparing practice with standards;
- describe how these difficulties might be avoided.

This stage compares the care which is actually being delivered with the care that the quality assurance group agreed should be delivered. This involves:-
- ❑ deciding **when** practice should be compared with standards;
- ❑ deciding **who** should be involved in comparing practice with standards;
- ❑ **comparing** observed practice with standards.

❑ Deciding when practice should be compared with standards

It takes time to appraise standards thoroughly and it would be time consuming, if not impossible, to appraise every standard on every occasion. A quality assurance group must decide when each standard is to be appraised and what aspects of it are to be appraised on a given occasion. The group specifies the:
- sub-topics;
- care groups;
- criteria
    - −structure
    - −process
    - −outcome

to be appraised on a particular date. This selection might be made:
- according to a plan;
- as problems emerge;
- at random.

Whichever of these tactics is adopted, it is good practice to ensure that each standard is appraised at least once a year.

Activity
Consider the following strategy:
Plan to appraise outcome criteria, and only appraise structure and process criteria in the event of poor outcomes.

Do you think that this is a sound strategy?

✎ Jot down a few reasons for your decision.

Some people follow the strategy suggested in the above activity. It saves time, **but** may lead to the group missing a situation where care could be improved if process and structure criteria were appraised. It is possible that care outcomes are good despite inadequate structure and process quality. Once dates are set, it is usual to make them widely known. This enables those who are involved or affected to plan accordingly. However, it also allows time for 'polishing bedrails' so that practice will appear better than it really is. This is partially offset by the benefits from thinking through what is involved in 'appearing better' !

❑ **Deciding who should be involved in comparing practice with standards**
So far, it has been assumed that the same quality group sets standards for a known setting and known care group, and appraises these standards. This might not be the case.

Activity
Consider the following list of people.

yes/no

- the group who wrote the standard
- senior administration or management
- colleagues within a peer review group
- quality consultants from outside the NHS
- members of a unit, district or regional audit committee

Against each, decide whether you think they could perform the appraisal.

✎ Jot down a few reasons for your answer.

Appraisal can be performed by any of the listed people. There are advantages and disadvantages associated with each choice. Some are given below.

- **Those who wrote the standard**
    advantages
    –thoroughly understand the standard.
    disadvantages
    –might be biased as they are so close to the situation.

- **Senior administration or management**
    advantages
    –bringing a wider perspective to appraisal.
    disadvantages
    –might be biased as they are ultimately responsible for quality;
    –might not be welcomed as assessors by professional staff.

- **Colleagues within a peer review group**
  advantages
  −work in a similar care setting to that being studied;
  −have the professional qualifications and experience to understand subtle nuances of care delivery;
  −usually have no vested interests as they do not work in the setting being appraised;
  −are acceptable to staff.
  disadvantages
  −may be biased in favour of colleagues with whom they have a close identification.

- **Quality consultants from outside the NHS**
  advantages
  −might be acceptable to clients and professional staff, depending upon their expertise;
  −do not have any institutional biases.
  disadvantages
  −might lack experience of the NHS and therefore be insensitive to the subtleties of care;
  −might be expensive compared with internal staff.

- **Members of a unit, district or regional audit committee**
  advantages
  −might comprise representatives from the groups already discussed;
  −might involve representatives from client pressure groups;
  −might involve clients or clients' relatives.
  disadvantages
  −professionals often doubt their capacity to 'really understand' what is happening in a particular care setting.

❑ Comparing observed practice with standards

The comparison of observed practice with standards is based on information collected through chosen measurement techniques. The comparison is aided by documenting the information in a structured format. Several formats are possible, but only one simple version is discussed here. The proforma for this is shown in diagram 14.

The initial steps have been specified in previous sections. They are to decide:
- which standards are to be considered;
- which care group is to be considered;
- what sample size is to be used;
- on what date the appraisal is to take place;
- who is to perform the appraisal;
- which type of appraisal is to be performed:
  −concurrent,
  −retrospective;
- which criteria are to be measured:
  −structure (S),
  −process (P),
  −outcome (O);
- how each criterion is be measured:
  −who or what will be observed,
  −who will be questioned,
  −which measurement technique will be used,
  −which records will be consulted.

Diagram 14   Proforma for Standard Appraisal

Topic:		Subtopic:					
Care Group:							
Standard Statement:							
Assessors:		Date of Appraisal					

S/P/O no.	CRITERIA (worded in question form)	MEASURED BY	WEIGHTING	YES	NO	N/A	Signature of assessor

for the standard:-

desired compliance rate =   observed compliance rate =

COMMENTS

e.g. Sample size (e.g. no. of clients appraised) ; reasons for results or N/A responses

The information from the initial steps is written on the appraisal form. The selected criteria are re-worded as questions and written in the second column.

The associated Structure, Process or Outcome number in column one allows cross-reference over different forms.

In column three, the assessor specifies the technique to be used to measure each criterion.

The next step is the completion of column four, 'Weighting'. The quality group decides the relative importance to be placed on each criterion to be measured. This relative importance is expressed as a weighting out of 100%. For example, if there are five criteria to be measured and all five criteria are equally important, then each criterion is assigned a weighting of

$$100/5 = 20\% .$$

However, if one criterion is deemed to be more important than the rest, then it is given a larger weighting, for example 40%. In this case, if the remaining four criteria are equally important they are assigned weightings of

$$(100 - 40)/4 = 15\% .$$

The remaining columns are completed by the assessor(s) during the appraisal. They show the assessor's decision as to whether each criterion is met (on the appraisal date)–Yes, No, or N/A (not applicable or exceptions).

When columns 1 through 7 are complete, the observed compliance rate is calculated. In its simplest form,

$$\text{observed compliance rate} = \frac{\text{Sum of (\textbf{WEIGHTING} \% x nos \textbf{YES})}}{\text{sample size}}$$

This observed compliance rate is compared with the desired compliance rate that is agreed by the quality group.

Space is allowed on the form for Comments. It is useful to know about any 'odd' occurrences. In particular, there may be some clients for whom a criterion does not immediately apply. In this case, the criterion is marked N/A and the reason could be noted under the Comments section of the form. Using simple arithmetic, this weighting may be discounted from the observed compliance rate.

Here is an example of a completed form, using the 'Safety' example standard from section 5.2.

Topic: Safety   **Subtopic:** Prevention of harm in the event of a fire

Care Group: All mobile patients on a 30 bedded surgical ward.

Standard Statement: That all mobile patients on the ward understand, and are aware of, the hospital fire policy, and can evacuate the premises in the event of a fire, thus avoiding danger.

Assessors: K. Brown   **Date of Appraisal:** 30.1.91

S/P/O no.	CRITERIA (worded in question form)	MEASURED BY	WEIGHTING	YES	NO	N/A	Signature of assessor
O1	Has the patient a fire information leaflet?	Ask Observe	10%	6	4		
O2	Does the patient understand the fire procedure?	Patient Questionnaire Ask	35%	9	1		
O3	Does the patient know where the fire equipment is on the ward?	Ask Observe	10%	5	5		
O4	Can a patient find their way to safety region?	Ask Observe	25%	9	1		
O5	Do the patients who smoke use the restricted smoking zone at all times?	Ask Observe	20%	4	6		

for the standard:-
     desired compliance rate = 100%   observed compliance rate = 73%
COMMENTS
10 patients appraised

In this example,

observed compliance rate = $\dfrac{(10 \times 6) + (35 \times 9) + (10 \times 5) + (25 \times 9) + (20 \times 4)}{10}$

❏ **Difficulties in comparing practice with standards**

Activity

✎ Jot down some reasons why the interpretation of quality assurance measurements might be difficult.

If :

- standards are appropriate;
- criteria are a precise index of standards;
- methods of measurement are appropriate;
- measurement techniques have been used accurately;
- contexts of measurement have been taken into account;

then there should be no difficulty in interpreting measurements.

But will this ever be the case?

There is always a difference between measurements taken and the conclusions which can justifiably be drawn from them. You have only to consider the different interpretations which politicians of opposing parties place on the same figures to realise that there are difficulties in going beyond the word 'therefore'.

Some of the problems in the measurement and appraisal of criteria and standards have been discussed in this and previous sections. It is good practice to try out a system before using it 'for real'. Such a dress rehearsal or trial run of the proposed appraisal is called piloting.

In these sections you have considered one approach to the appraisal of standards. You have now completed the first half of the quality wheel. You may wish to assess your understanding of the material by working through the following questions.

Self-assessment Question 10

✎ Complete the 'Summary of Quality Appraisal' by inserting into the spaces provided the eight appropriate words from the list given below.

Wordlist

clients	extensive	managers	practitioners	subjective
concurrent	idealised	objective	results	topic
criteria	inexpensive	observed	small	unbiased
effective	inexperienced	outcome	statements	written

Summary of Quality Appraisal

Quality appraisal is the first process in any quality assurance initiative. It is followed by quality action. Quality appraisal involves setting up a QA group; setting and agreeing standards; selecting and using measurement techniques; and, comparing _____$_1$ practice with standards.

A quality assurance group usually has between four and ten members, one of whom is an _____$_2$ leader. Group meetings should last no longer than 1 1/2 hours and be conducted around a clear agenda.

The quality assurance group selects a _____$_3$ and then subtopics for the development of standards. Each standard is written for a defined set of _____$_4$ or care group and specifies a desirable, acceptable and achievable level of care. Once a standard has been written, _____$_5$ are prepared which specify clearly and precisely the levels of performance which have to be achieved to satisfy the standard. Donabedian identified three types of criteria: structure, process and _____$_6$. Criteria should be checked for suitability against the AMOUR principle.

It is important when setting standards and establishing criteria to consider when and how they will be monitored. Appraisal of care may be _____$_7$ or retrospective. Various measurement techniques can be used including assessment/audit, interviews, questionnaires and conferences.

The final step in quality appraisal is to use selected measurement techniques to compare observed practice with standards. It is important to select an _____$_8$ sample to assess and to consider carefully who performs the appraisal.

Self-assessment Question 11

For each of the following statements, decide whether it is true or false.

✎ Circle your answer.

1) The larger the size of the quality assurance group the more successful the quality assurance initiative.

True/False

2) Standards should be written on subtopics that are within the quality assurance group's area of responsibility.

True/False

3) Outcome criteria specify the end results of care.

True/False

4) A selected measurement technique must be suitable for the care group.

True/False

5) A quality assurance group always appraises its own standards.

True/False

Self-assessment Question 12

Refer to process criterion 6 of example standard 2 in section 2.4 :
The occupational therapist discusses with the client, carers and the support services methods of overcoming identified problem areas.

a) How many points are covered in this one criterion?

b) Word this criterion in question form.

Self-assessment Question 13

The following information is taken from a standard appraisal form:

S/P/O no.	WEIGHTING	YES	NO
P2	10%	6	2
P4	10%	8	0
S1	15%	7	1
S2	15%	8	0
O2	25%	7	1
O3	25%	6	2

✎ If 8 patients were appraised, calculate the observed compliance rate.

Solutions to self-assessment questions

Solution to Self-assessment Question 10

space	word
1	observed
2	effective
3	topic
4	clients
5	criteria
6	outcome
7	concurrent
8	unbiased

Solution to Self-assessment Question 11

1) False

The success of a quality assurance initiative is not guaranteed when the group membership is large (more than ten). Such a group may be representative of clients, practitioners, managers and others likely to be affected by the standard. However, agreement may be difficult to achieve and discussions may become very time-consuming. A small group (two to four members) is often sufficient, depending upon the scope of the intended quality assurance initiative. It is certainly beneficial to have more than one member as this facilitates the generation, sharing and discussion of ideas.

2) True

Standards should be written on subtopics that are within the quality assurance group's area of responsibility. This influences the promotion of 'ownership' of a standard by those who use it. It also implies that a standard is written by people with the relevant knowledge and insight. Further, as discussed in the following sections on quality action, it facilitates the introduction of any necessary change.

3) True

Outcome criteria specify the end results of care. Most outcome criteria are concerned with the effects of care upon clients and, therefore, are more important than structure and process criteria. Satisfying structure and process criteria does not guarantee the satisfaction of outcome criteria. Outcome criteria can be satisfied when structure or process criteria are not.

4) True

A selected measurement technique must be suitable for the care group. For example, client interviews would be unsuitable for those with senile dementia, or for those in a coma.

5) False

A standard can be appraised by:
   those who wrote it;
   senior administration or management;
   colleagues within a peer review group;
   quality consultants from outside the NHS;
   members of a unit, district or regional audit committee.

Solution to Self-assessment Question 12

a) Three points are covered by the criterion. The occupational therapist discusses methods of overcoming identified problem areas with:
> 1. the clients;
> 2. the carers;
> 3. the support services.

It may be better practice to write criteria that contain only one point.

b) There will be three associated questions:

Has the occupational therapist discussed methods of overcoming identified problem areas with the client?

Has the occupational therapist discussed methods of overcoming identified problem areas with the carers?

Has the occupational therapist discussed methods of overcoming identified problem areas with the support services?

Different measurement techniques may be applicable in each case.

Solution to Self-assessment Question 13

Observed compliance rate = sum of(WEIGHTING % x nos YES) / (sample size)

sum of (WEIGHTING % x nos YES) =	10x6 + 10x8 + 15x7 + 15x8 + 25x7 + 25x6
=	60 + 80 + 105 + 120 + 175 + 150
=	690
sample size =	8
Observed compliance rate =	690 / 8
=	86%

6   The Steps in Quality Action

Objectives:
By the end of this section you will be able to:
- describe each of the steps involved in quality action;
- discuss review of standards.

To achieve the first objective we will work through the stages shown in diagram 15.

Diagram 15   Quality Action

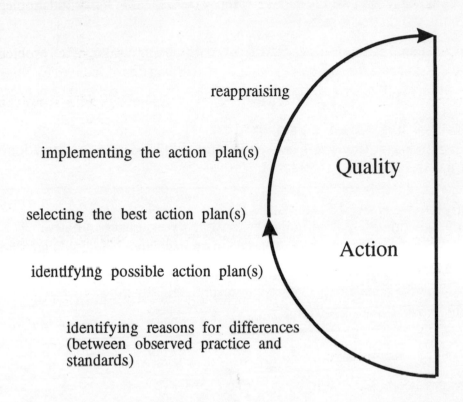

reappraising

implementing the action plan(s)

selecting the best action plan(s)

identifying possible action plan(s)

identifying reasons for differences (between observed practice and standards)

Quality

Action

6.1 Identifying reasons for differences
(between observed practice and standards)

Objectives:
By the end of this section you will be able to:
- discuss the possible differences between observed practice and standards;
- state reasons for reviewing membership of a quality assurance group at this stage;
- name one method for identifying reasons for any quality gaps;
- discuss ways of communicating information to colleagues.

When all the steps in quality appraisal are complete, the quality assurance group is ready to tackle quality action. This is an essential part of quality assurance. There is no point in collecting information if it is not used to instigate action to improve quality of care.

Action is planned in response to the comparison of observed practice with a standard. Standards are difficult to set with precision and measurement is imperfect, so it is prudent to consider all measurements carefully before any action is discussed. Were the measures really valid, or were there special circumstances that affected the results? If there is any doubt, it may be necessary to re-appraise the standard.

Once the measurements are considered to be sound, then the process of quality action can begin. The quality assurance group is faced with two possible situations for each standard appraised:
- ❏ observed practice meets or exceeds the standard;
- ❏ observed practice falls short of the standard.

In either case the quality assurance group will want to discuss the results.

❏ Observed practice meets or exceeds the standard

Firstly, everyone involved should be congratulated. Even a little praise can boost morale.

Then, the quality assurance group must reconsider the situation to glean information to help in the process of continuous quality improvement. For example:-

Has observed practice consistently met or exceeded the standard on previous appraisals? If so, then maybe the standard should be reviewed.

Is the observed compliance rate higher than on previous appraisals? If so, then query what changes have been made to procedures and/or resources that might account for this. Could this have implications with regard to other aspects of care (either beneficial or detrimental)?

❏ Observed practice falls short of the standard

In this situation where a quality gap has been identified, goodwill and motivation for quality improvement are very important.

Activity

Imagine that your work group is participating in a quality assurance initiative. The observed practice is found to fall short of the standard in an area where you are directly involved.

✎ Jot down some thoughts on how you might react to this situation.

✎ Jot down some ways you could be informed about it, and say which of them you would prefer.

Attempts at change are doomed unless the results of quality appraisal are perceived as well-intentioned, constructive feedback. Communication should be:
- ● specific,
    - –it is easier to understand ' there are no fire extinguishers' than 'safety apparatus is inadequate';
- ● as positive as possible,
    - –phrase the information so that no criticism and no blame is implied and begin with good points from the appraisal;
- ● confidential,
    - –if specific individuals or groups are identified as contributing to the poor compliance rate, restrict the information to an appropriate sub-group.

All members of a quality assurance group, indeed everyone involved in a quality assurance initiative, need to respond to this situation with a positive attitude. There is nothing to be gained either by looking for a scapegoat or by rushing into poorly planned action.

Before discussing any action, it is important to clarify the area of work or aspect of care that does not satisfy the standard. The next task is to determine possible reasons for this. It is worth asking:

- Has observed practice consistently fallen short of the standard on previous appraisals? Why?

- Is the observed compliance rate lower than on previous appraisals? Why?

(You may have suggested asking questions concerning 'where' and 'why' in your response to the activity above). In this and many other situations, a useful and powerful technique for generating possible solutions is 'brainstorming'.

- **Brainstorming**

    Brainstorming is a commonly used group activity used to generate ideas. To achieve a wide view, it is suggested that the group involves between five to twelve people, including:

    —experts;
    —semi-experts;
    —practitioners;
    —support staff;

    in the area under consideration.

    The quality assurance group might already have this composition. If not, it may be helpful to change the membership for this stage.

    One person is elected as session leader, perhaps the chairperson of the quality assurance group. The session leader has a very important task. This person must:

    —keep enthusiasm and intensity high;
    —encourage everyone to participate;
    —collect as many ideas as possible by going repeatedly around the group;
    —ask each person, in turn, to contribute an idea (a person may 'pass');
    —allow no comment (supportive or adverse) about ideas while they are being generated;
    —record the group's ideas on a clipboard so that everyone can see them;
    —when everyone 'passes' encourage the group to proceed to judge the generated ideas.

    For their part, team members:

    —generate as many ideas as possible;
    —contribute all their ideas (no matter how 'extreme' or 'silly');
    —suspend judgement upon the ideas of others;
    —build upon the ideas of others.

    The leader then helps the group to agree which of the proposed reasons seem most plausible.

By the end of this step, the quality assurance group has a list of the most plausible reasons for the quality gap and is now ready to identify action plans.

6.2 Identifying possible action plan(s)

> **Objectives**
> By the end of this section you will be able to:
> - state a reason for reviewing membership of a quality assurance group at this stage;
> - state a reason why management might be represented on the quality assurance group;
> - discuss the generation of action plans.

During the previous step on the quality wheel, plausible reasons were identified for observed practice falling short of standards. These reasons are the starting point from which action plans are identified to improve quality so that standards can be achieved.

Another brainstorming session may be used to generate a set of possible action plans. These plans must be:
- realistic;
- acceptable to individuals and groups who will be affected by agreed changes;
- acceptable to management.

These conditions influence the membership of the quality assurance group. It is important to have:
- representatives of those who will be affected by agreed changes;
- management representatives with some authority to approve or ease the implementation of action plans.

This revised group is referred to as the action group.

By the end of this step, the group has a list of the most plausible action plans and is now ready to select a suitable one.

6.3 Selecting the best action plan(s)

Objectives
By the end of this section you will be able to:
- list questions that an action group should consider before selecting a plan;
- comment on the relationship between quality action and cost effectiveness.

Selecting an action plan involves examining the proposed plans for desirability and feasibility. As part of this exercise, for each suggested plan the action group considers questions such as:
- Is the proposed action realistic within available resources?
- Is it capable of solving the problem(s) in a reasonable time?
- Is it capable of solving the problem(s) with reasonable effort?
- Is it acceptable to senior management?
- Is it acceptable to colleagues?
- Is it within existing organisational policy guidelines?
- Who and what is likely to be affected by its implementation?
- Are suitable, enthusiastic personnel available to take charge of it?
- Are the anticipated results of the action measurable? (The original criteria may be applicable here).
- Will it cost a lot to implement compared with what it should achieve?

Activity

✎ Jot down some reasons why you think it is important to consider costs.

Answering the suggested questions is not an easy task. Further, it is obvious that they lead to yet more questions that must be considered before a decision is taken. However, this investigative process is made easier when the action group has appropriate members, as discussed at the previous stage.

Decisions made during discussions on costs and resources will have implications for many of the questions. It is, therefore, important that the availability of resources and the costs of implementing plans are taken into account during the selection procedure. For example, suppose that practitioners' lack of skill or knowledge is identified as a plausible reason for a standard not being met. A possible solution could be a series of in-service study days. However, there are several reasons why this plan might be unrealistic, including:
- the cost of taking practitioners out of the care setting for long periods of study is unacceptable,
    - −cost in monetary terms,
    - −cost in terms of loss of care available to clients;
- there are insufficient tutorial staff to cover the training.

Donabedian (1986) proposed three points to consider when viewing quality in relation to costs:
- quality costs money;
- money does not necessarily buy quality;
- some improvements in quality are not worth the added cost.

A rejoinder to this last point is:
- continuing 'poor' quality service may be even more expensive in the long run.

The cost implications of effecting improvement and of continuing with 'poor' quality should both be set out. It is also vital that the action group explores possible consequences for the quality of care elsewhere in the system. Robbing Peter to pay Paul is not good quality action.

When the final choice is made, it should be agreed by:
- everyone directly affected by the change;
- management;
- the action group.

The actual action plan should specify:
- ❏ a clear schedule;
- ❏ the time it will take to carry out each step;
- ❏ dates for progress reports;
- ❏ dates for publicity initiatives;
- ❏ a final completion date;
- ❏ a date for reappraisal of the standard;
- ❏ a date for review of the standard.

Upon completion of this step, the action group has selected a 'best' plan of action. The next stage is to implement the plan.

6.4 Implementing the action plan(s)

Objectives:
By the end of this section you will be able to:
- list three approaches to implementing change;
- outline a strategy for communication about change;
- outline the role of an 'action coordinator';
- discuss the evaluation of action plans.

In the previous stage, the action group selected an action plan and identified who was likely to be affected by it. The quality action group is now ready to prepare people for change and to implement the action plan.

Traditionally, change is a difficult business. However carefully action plans are formed, actually putting them into operation can create disruption and stress. This section discusses some general principles of organisational change and offers specific guidance for implementing changes associated with the assurance of quality.

The health service is made up of diverse individuals doing diverse jobs in diverse settings. In such a large organisation, changing the routine activities of any individual in any setting has some impact, however small, on all of the others. As seen in unit one, people affected include health care professionals, managers, administrators, support workers, voluntary workers, clients, their families and neighbours. Everyone must be willing to accept change if the quality of health care is to be continually improved. A quality assurance initiative is a fruitless exercise if people or systems are not open to change.

Activity
Decide which of the following approaches to change is the most likely to encourage enthusiastic involvement:
- ❑ telling people that the change will be a good thing and detailing benefits for the organisation;
- ❑ telling people they must change and implying it could be the worse for them if they don't;
- ❑ involving people in sorting out what the change will mean for them and offering them help in implementing it.

✎ Jot down some reasons for your choice.

You probably noted that people will respond more positively if they know exactly what change is proposed and, more importantly, why. It should be emphasised that the intention is to improve the quality of care given to clients and not merely to initiate change for its own sake.

You might feel that some element of each of the above approaches is helpful. The best balance between them will depend upon the type of change involved and the type of organisation in which it is to be implemented.

The third approach is probably both the most difficult to execute and the one most likely to succeed! It is the only one likely to foster long-lasting change. Using this approach in health care means that staff and clients must be:

- given regular information updates;
- encouraged to put forward their points of view;
- listened to;
- allowed to challenge ideas;
- thoroughly involved in the change process.

People who are kept up to date with the proceedings of the quality assurance/action group are more prepared to accept change. **Good communication is an essential prerequisite of change**.

There is another important advantage of the third approach. Discussion and feedback from a wide range of colleagues could reveal a flaw in the 'best' action plan that has not been taken into account. This could mean that the action group has to reconsider other possible action plans.

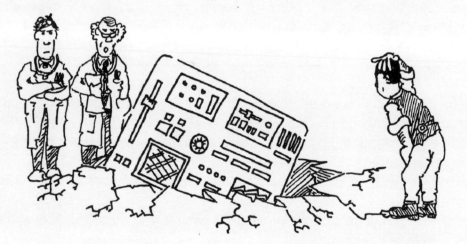

'I could have told you that you couldn't shift it to this room'

Activity

Find out what methods are used to communicate quality action in your work place.

✎ Jot down some advantages and disadvantages of each in your opinion.

If none are in evidence, jot down a few ideas why you think that this is so.

You might have found some of the following methods in use:

- ❑ organising meetings with colleagues, updating them on standard setting and appraisal, discussing any proposed action strategies with them;
- ❑ circulating minutes from action group meetings to relevant people;
- ❑ making personal contact with people likely to be affected by the action plan;
- ❑ producing a quality newsletter or contributing to a more general one;
- ❑ organising a quality notice board in a prominent place;
- ❑ running and reporting on quality competitions.

Communicating the action plan is not enough to ensure that action is carried out. When it comes to actually getting something done, it is helpful to identify one individual whose responsibility it is to make sure that progress takes place. This individual is referred to as an 'action coordinator'.

Activity

Think of an individual who might make a good action coordinator in your own care setting.

✎ Jot down some personal traits that led you to choose this person.

You have probably included characteristics such as possessing:

- • knowledge appropriate to the action to be taken;
- • skills appropriate to the action to be taken;
- • good social skills (e.g. leadership, ability to persuade and motivate colleagues);
- • a good network of contacts with practitioners, management and other relevant groups;
- • clinical credibility.

Whether the action coordinator is someone with senior or junior status within the organisation depends upon the changes proposed. But where these will directly affect clinical practice then the coordinator must be acceptable to the relevant clinicians.

In certain circumstances help is needed from outside the organisation. For example, if the appraisal highlighted the fact that clinical staff were using some specialised equipment incorrectly, then an external expert might provide relevant training. Likewise if the appraisal showed that the arrangement of rooms was therapeutically inadequate, then an architect's help might be sought.

With or without outside help, the action coordinator is responsible for:
- setting a schedule for change;
- strict monitoring of deadlines,
   −issuing periodic reminders helps to galvanise people into action and keep them involved;
- feedback of progress reports,
   −determining frequency of progress reports to departmental heads, practitioners, action group,
   −publicising dates when feedback reports should appear;
- agreement that completion of the action has actually taken place;
- making sure that communication is flowing smoothly;
- smoothing out disputes.

To formally determine the success of an action plan, a reappraisal of the standard is necessary.

6.5 Reappraising

Objective:

By the end of this section you will be able to:

● discuss some aspects of reappraising a standard.

Reappraisal entails re-assessing a standard using the same criteria and measurement techniques as in the original appraisal. As soon as the action initiatives seem to be properly in place, a reappraisal should confirm the beneficial effects (or otherwise) of the action taken. Some caution should be exercised however, since reappraising a standard too soon after implementing action can have the effect of discouraging colleagues who have not had an opportunity to consolidate new activities.

If the action has not resulted in the standard being met, then the group must initiate another action plan and another reappraisal in pursuit of improvement. In some instances, observed practice consistently falls short of the standard, in which case it is time that the standard was reviewed.

Reappraisal is the last step on the quality wheel. We have now discussed all the steps in quality appraisal and quality action. A further important task for the quality assurance group to perform is the review of standards.

6.6 Reviewing standards

Objective:
By the end of this section you will be able to:
- describe some aspects of reviewing standards.

From time to time (probably once per year) the quality assurance group should undertake an overall review of the standards that they have set and agreed. In this review, members of the group discuss the results of quality appraisals and reappraisals and determine appropriate action to be taken about the standards themselves.

For example, difficulties might be highlighted with measurement techniques or other aspects of appraisal of a particular standard. The group could decide to rewrite the standard to be more explicit, or to rewrite its criteria, or to specify the use of different measurement techniques. For another standard, records might show that the standard has been met consistently. Here the group could try to improve quality by increasing the desired compliance rate, or by writing more demanding requirements into the criteria. On the other hand, the group might decide that it is time to develop a new standard or even to consider a new topic. That is, to go round the wheel again. On this occasion however, some steps might be unnecessary and others might be accomplished more quickly.

In these sections you have considered approaches to quality action. You have now completed the second half of the quality wheel. You may wish to assess your understanding of the material by working through the following questions.

Self-assessment Question 14

✎ Complete the 'Summary of Quality Action' by inserting into the spaces provided the eight appropriate words from the list given below.

Wordlist

capable	costs	generate	realistic	responsibility
change	desirability	inexpensive	reappraisal	review
confidential	excuses	list	reasons	select
coordinator	expert	quick	resources	successful

Summary of Quality Action

Quality action follows quality appraisal and is an essential part of quality assurance. Action is planned in response to the comparison of observed practice with a standard. There are two possible situations for each standard appraised; observed practice either exceeds or falls short of the standard. In the latter case, practitioners need to be informed of the results in a manner that is specific, as positive as possible and _____ $_1$. The quality assurance group then seeks to identify _____ $_2$ for the shortfall, perhaps using a technique such as brainstorming to _____ $_3$ possible solutions. The identified plausible reasons form the starting point from which action plans are created to improve quality so that standards can be achieved. Action plans must be _____ $_4$, be acceptable to individuals and groups who will be affected by agreed changes, and be acceptable to management. It may be necessary to review membership of the quality assurance group at this stage.

The quality action group examines the proposed plans for _____ $_5$ and feasibility and selects a best action plan. It is important that the availability of _____ $_6$ and the costs of implementing plans are taken into account during the selection procedure. The implementation of the selected plan is managed by an action _____ $_7$, who ensures that the plan is actually carried out, that target dates are met and that progress reports are published. Once the action plan has been implemented, its success is evaluated through a _____ $_8$ of the standard.

From time to time, the quality assurance group should undertake an overall review of the standards that they have set and agreed. This may result in amending some standards, or in developing new standards.

Self-assessment Question 15

For each of the following statements, decide whether it is true or false.

✎ Circle your answer.

1) During a brainstorming session, ideas are not judged until as many ideas as possible have been generated.

True/False

2) Management representatives should not be included in the quality action group as they may impede open discussion.

True/False

3) The most effective way of implementing change is to involve the people affected by the change and to help them to implement it.

True/False

4) A good action coordinator will always be someone in a senior position in the care setting.

True/False

Self-assessment Question 16

✎ State why quality action is an essential part of any quality assurance initiative.

Solutions to self-assessment questions

Solution to Self-assessment Question 14

space	word
1	confidential
2	reasons
3	generate
4	realistic
5	desirability
6	resources
7	coordinator
8	reappraisal

Solutions to questions 15 and 16 are given on page 102

Solution to Self-assessment Question 15

1)   True

During a brainstorming session as many ideas as possible are collected before each idea is discussed and judged. This encourages everyone to contribute. It also allows unlikely ideas to be expressed that after group discussion may lead to the generation of imaginative, feasible plans.

2)   False

If management is committed to quality improvement then their representatives will encourage open discussions in the action group. Also, management representatives with some authority may be able to approve or ease the implementation of action plans.

3)   True

The most effective way of implementing change is to involve the people affected by the change and to help them to implement it. Several reasons for the likely success of this approach were given in section 6.4 .

4)   False

The coordinator may be someone with senior or junior status within the organisation, or someone from outside the organisation. This depends upon the changes proposed. Some desirable characteristics of an action coordinator were given in section 6.4.

Solution to Self-assessment Question 16

Quality action is an essential process, it uses the information gained from quality appraisal to initiate improvement in the quality of care/service. There is no point collecting information if it not used. Quality assurance is about improving quality for the client.

FOLLOWING THE STEPS

104

7 Introduction to Following the Steps : A Clinical Scenario

In unit one Understanding Quality, you met the concepts of quality and quality assurance. You discovered who is interested in quality and how quality assurance developed in the health service. Also in that unit you were introduced to the setting of standards.

In unit two you explored the steps involved in assessing and improving quality. These were divided into quality appraisal steps and quality action steps.

In this unit you will be given the opportunity to use what you have learned in the previous two units. You will be given an everyday clinical scenario in which to apply the steps on the quality wheel.

Objective
By the end of this unit you will have:
- used the information gained in units one and two in a hypothetical clinical scenario.

7.1 The scenario

In this section we describe a clinical setting. We are assuming that most of our readers have some familiarity with hospital care although we realise that many work in other settings.

❑ Quality system
A quality strategy exists at the Regional level. At the District and Unit levels, designated individuals are responsible for quality including setting up quality systems. A wide variety of quality initiatives are taking place including client satisfaction surveys, quality circles and standard setting. The purchaser and provider contract system has increased the importance of clear quality standards. Some surgeons and physicians are also involved in medical audits. All health professions in your Unit of Management are being encouraged to develop quality assurance activities.

❑ Client care setting
You are a health professional working in the acute medical ward of a modern medium sized (300-bedded) general hospital. The Medical Ward itself has 24 beds arranged in cubicles of four and a small day room.

A team of health care professionals including doctors, nurses and professions allied to medicine is available in the clinical setting. There are facilities within the hospital for both in- and out-patient care.

❑ Clients
The clients on the ward include people with the following health care problems:

- cardio-respiratory;
- neurological;
- metabolic.

For the purpose of this exercise we suggest that you select clients from the neurological group.

7.2 Writing the standard

□ **Topic**

For this exercise we have selected rehabilitation as the topic area. You may wish to refer back to page 62, section 5.2 to review what is involved in choosing a topic.

□ **Subtopic**

Here are a few subtopics which you could use in relation to the topic rehabilitation:

1. dressing
2. postural balance
3. mobilising
4. information giving.

Activity

Add another four possible subtopics to this list, focusing on areas with which you would be directly involved.

5._____
6._____
7._____
8._____

For now we suggest that you select mobilising as the subtopic. At this point, if you are feeling confident, you may choose to involve other health care professionals in the activity–many would have a knowledge and interest in this subtopic area.

□ **Care group**

Care groups to which a neurological client might belong include:

● newly admitted clients following cerebro-vascular accidents (CVA);
● clients ready for discharge following CVA;
● clients who have Parkinson's disease;
● clients who have multiple sclerosis.

For now consider the second client group identified above.

An example of a client who would fit into this group is Mr. George Smith, a 56 year-old, self-employed plumber who works with his son in the family firm. Mr. Smith lives at home with his wife who is a full-time housewife. Their home is a detached two-storey house in the suburbs of a large city. The family company is run from home and before his illness Mr. Smith also worked enthusiastically in their large garden. The son is married and lives close by with his young family.

Six weeks ago Mr. Smith suffered a right cerebro-vascular accident resulting in a dense left hemiplegia. Fortunately, his speech and vision were not affected.

❏ Standard statement

Activity

Refer back to page 63, section 5.2 where the writing of standard statements was discussed.

✎ Now write a standard statement for the specified care group of clients ready for discharge following CVA:

Topic: Rehabilitation
Subtopic: Mobilising
Care Group: Clients ready for discharge following CVA
Standard Statement:

Remember, your statement will probably be a short quality oriented sentence related to your subtopic and care group (i.e. mobilising clients who are ready for discharge following CVA). Refer back to the checklist on page 63, section 5.2 to help you in this task. This specified that a standard statement should:

- be clearly written;
- address an agreed topic;
- pertain to an agreed care group;
- be acceptable to relevant colleagues.

❏ Criteria

Now that you have your standard statement, think about the associated structure, process and outcome criteria that will allow you to judge when the standard has or has not been met.

✎ For now write three structure, three process and two outcome criteria.

Topic: Rehabilitation
Subtopic: Mobilising
Care Group: Clients ready for discharge following CVA
Standard Statement:

No.	Structure	No.	Process	No.	Outcome
1)		1)		1)	
2)		2)		2)	
3)		3)			

Remember your criteria must satisfy the AMOUR principle (page 66, section 5.3). That is, criteria should be:

- **A**chievable;
- **M**easurable;
- **O**bservable;
- **U**nderstandable;
- **R**easonable.

Now that you have prepared your standard statement and identified the criteria, check that the criteria are compatible with the statement. You may wish to return to the standard statement and refine it based on the criteria that you have written.

You can now move on to identifying suitable measurement techniques.

7.3 Measurement techniques

Activity

Obviously, you could measure all of the criteria that you have written. For this exercise only, choose four criteria, at least one from each of the categories structure, process and outcome.

✎ Word these chosen criteria in question form and enter this information on the following form:

Topic: Rehabilitation   **Subtopic:** Mobilising

Care Group: Clients ready for discharge following CVA

Standard Statement:

Assessors: **Date of Appraisal**

S/P/O no.	CRITERIA (worded in question form)	MEASURED BY	WEIGHTING	YES	NO	N/A	Signature of assessor
				1	4		
				3	2		
				5	0		
				3	2		

for the standard:-

desired compliance rate = 100%   observed compliance rate =

COMMENTS
sample size 5 clients

Having rewritten your criteria in question form, move on and identify how each will be measured. Try to include a variety of measurement techniques and check that you can justify your choices. You may find pages 70 to 75, section 5.3 helpful; the following measurement techniques were discussed there:
- assessment/audit;
- interviews;
- questionnaires;
- conferences;
- direct observation.

Now consider the weighting you would allocate to each of the criteria you have chosen to appraise. If each of the four criteria have equal importance, give each a weighting of 25%. If you consider some criteria to be more important than others then reflect this in your weightings.

❑ Calculating observed compliance rate

Using the above form you will see that a sample of five clients has been taken from the care group. We have entered hypothetical figures to indicate whether the criteria have been met or not for these five clients.

We have decided that for this standard a 100% compliance rate is desired.

In this exercise, we have ensured that 100% compliance has not been reached.

The next stage is to identify the reasons for this difference between observed and desired compliance rates—that is the observed 'quality gap'.

110

7.4 Quality action

❏ Reasons for differences

> **Activity**
>
> Think about possible reasons why the 'quality gap' has occurred. Refer to the 'NO' column on the appraisal form and brainstorm possible reasons for these 'NO' responses.
>
> ✎ Jot down a few of these reasons

❏ Action plans

By now you will have identified some possible reasons for the 'quality gap'.

> **Activity**
>
> ✎ Suggest three plans of action to either narrow or close the quality gap for one of the appraised criteria where there is a predominantly 'NO' response.
>
> **Criteria:**
>
> **Possible action plans**
>
> I
>
> II
>
> III

❏ Select the best action plan

Check each of your suggested action plans for desirability and feasibility by referring to the questions listed on page 91, section 6.3.

Activity

These questions are rephrased below as statements. For each of the three proposed action plans,

✎ jot down a mark from 1 (strong disagreement) to 5 (high agreement) against each statement:

Statement	Action plan		
	I	**II**	**III**
The proposed action is realistic within available resources	—	—	—
It is capable of solving the problem(s) in a reasonable time	—	—	—
It is capable of solving the problem(s) with reasonable effort	—	—	—
It is acceptable to senior management	—	—	—
It is acceptable to colleagues	—	—	—
It is within existing organisational policy guidelines	—	—	—
Suitable, enthusiastic personnel are available to take charge of it	—	—	—
The anticipated results of the action are measurable	—	—	—
It will not cost a lot to implement compared with what it should achieve	—	—	—

Sum these marks for each plan to obtain a ranking of the proposed plans.

Remember to consider the question:

> 'Who and what is likely to be affected by its implementation?'

Answers to this could change the ranking obtained above.

Activity

Select one of the proposed action plans for implementation.

❏ Implementing the action plan

In the real clinical situation you would now implement your chosen action plan and then reappraise its success at a given date.

You have now completed the steps on the quality wheel.

Activity

If you have worked through this exercise on your own, it may be beneficial to return to the subtopic list on page 106 and repeat the exercise with one or more colleagues.

Equally, if you have progressed through the exercise as a member of a group, you may find that repeating the exercise with a different subtopic will be constructive.

You should now be in a position to contribute to quality assurance initiatives. These may be with other health professionals, clients and their families, in hospital and non-hospital settings.

What is your next step?

LOOKING TO THE FUTURE

8 Aims and Objectives Reviewed

Objective:
By the end of this unit you will:
- have identified what you have achieved by studying this workbook.

You will recall from page 1 that our aims for this workbook were:

- to provide an overview of quality assurance for you, the health care professional;
- to sketch the historical background to quality assurance development;
- to increase your understanding and appreciation of quality assurance in your professional field;
- to encourage your enthusiastic participation in quality assurance programmes;
- to introduce some quality assurance techniques appropriate to your professional work as a member of a multi-disciplinary team.

In unit one, we provided an overview of quality assurance and traced its historical development. In unit two we presented a guide to the steps involved in a quality assurance initiative and incorporated some techniques that are suitable for use by a multi-disciplinary health care team. We hope that these units have increased your understanding and appreciation of quality assurance in your professional field.

In unit three we helped you to participate in a quality assurance initiative in a hypothetical health care setting. We cannot be certain but we would like to think that this, along with the other units, has encouraged your enthusiastic, confident participation in real quality assurance programmes in your future practice.

We have thus monitored the extent to which we have achieved the underlying objectives for this workbook. You should now monitor the extent to which you have met your own objectives.

Activity

✎ Jot down what you have achieved by studying this workbook.

Now compare practice with standards by looking back at what you hoped to achieve when you completed the box on page 1.

You have now reached the end of this workbook. We hope that you have enjoyed working through it.

What is your next step?

Initially, you may wish to progress by joining an existing quality assurance group with experienced members, or one of the quality assurance networks suggested in section 3.5. This will depend upon what quality assurance initiatives are taking place in your work setting. Alternatively, you may wish to generate small, local initiatives. Whatever your choice, we wish you well in the pursuit of quality care.

GLOSSARY OF TERMS

Acceptable   a service provision that satisfies the reasonable expectations of the patient, provider and society.

Accessible   a service provision not compromised by undue limits of time, distance or cost.

Accountability   the state of being answerable for one's decisions and actions. Accountability cannot be delegated.

Accreditation   the process by which an agency or organisation evaluates and recognises a programme of study or an institution as meeting predetermined standards.

Adequacy   the allocation of activities and resources in manner and quantity sufficient to permit the achievement of desired objectives.

Appraisal   the formulating, achieving agreement upon and monitoring of standards.

Approachable   allows open communication with clients, peers and others.

Appropriate   provision of a service or procedure that the population or an individual requires.

Assessment   the thorough study of a known or suspected problem in quality of care, designed to define causes and necessary action to correct the problem.

Assurance   a statement or assertion intended to inspire confidence, pledge or promise of support, freedom from doubt, making sure.

Audit   a methodical review or investigation of resources and activities.

Autonomy   the right to self-directed professional judgement and treatment planning.

Caring   (1) providing for the physical and psychological needs of a client in a therapeutic environment;
(2) an holistic empathetic approach to service provision.

Client   denotes the participant in care, who in some settings may be called the patient/customer/recipient of care.

Committed   allegiance to given professional values and standards of care and service.

Communication   exchange of information, ideas or feelings.

Competence   presence of necessary knowledge, skills and personal attitudes to allow for the performance of professional tasks.

Comprehensive   service offering a wide range of abilities and specialities.

Contract   a written agreement by a provider to provide a service within given stipulations to a purchaser.

Cost-effective	able to achieve the intended objective(s) with the optimum use of resources.
Criteria	(1) professionally developed statements of optimal health care structure, process, or outcome; (2) descriptive statements which are measurable and which reflect the intent of a standard in terms of performance, behaviour, circumstances or clinical states. A number of criteria may be developed for each standard.
Economic	planned use of resources to avoid unnecessary waste.
Effective	able to achieve the intended objective(s) for the individual or the population.
Efficacy	the benefit or utility to the individual of the services, treatment regimen, drug, preventive or control measure advocated or applied.
Efficiency	the ratio between the result that might be achieved through the expenditure of a specified amount of resources and the result that might be achieved through a minimum of expenditure.
Equity	fairness, impartiality.
Ethical	observes clients' rights and professional codes of conduct.
Evaluation	the systematic and scientific process of determining the extent to which an action or sets of actions were successful in the achievement of predetermined objectives.
Expert	has extensive skill or knowledge in a particular field.
Holistic	an approach to care which takes account of the needs of whole individuals, in relation to their physical, psychological, social, intellectual and spiritual states.
Monitoring	the ongoing measurements of a variety of indicators of health care quality to identify potential problems.
Objective	a measurable state that is expected to exist at a predetermined place and time as a result of the application of procedures and resources.
Outcome	(1) the results of health care activity described in terms of the effect on clients; (2) a change in the current and future health status of the client that can be attributed to antecedent health care.
Peer	a person who has equal standing with another person in a particular social context; especially concerns rank, status, education or authority.
Peer review	(1) the activities of an individual or group are subjected to scrutiny by another individual or group with comparable training and experience, who is therefore competent to draw conclusions about activities or performance; (2) the evaluation of quality of performance of individuals or groups by peers using established criteria in a defined or given situation.
Philosophy	a set of values and beliefs which guides thoughts and actions.

Policy   a statement representing a course of action adopted by, or on behalf of, an organisation and its members.

Process   the treatment management activities of health care professionals, such as clinical assessment, treatment and preventative care, as well as documentation and other related activities.

Purchaser-Provider System
          through contracts Purchasers (for example Health Authorities) will buy the services they need for their population, paying the Provider for that service.

Quality   (1) degree or standard of excellence; a distinguishing characteristic or attribute; in health care includes such aspects as access, relevance, effectiveness, equity, efficiency, economy, social acceptability;
          (2) the totality of features and characteristics of a product or service that bear on its ability to satisfy a given need;
          (3) a level of excellence identified by an agreed standard, and reflecting achievable and desirable objectives based on the values of those who set the standard;

          'A product has a good quality if it is meeting the standards that have been set before the evaluation took place.'   Van Maanen (1979)

          'The adherence to standards and criteria that are based on current knowledge and sound experience.'   Sanazaro (1986)

Quality assessment
          the measurement of provision against expectations.

Quality assurance
          (1) a process in which achievable and desirable levels of quality are described, the extent to which these levels are achieved and action taken to enable them to be reached is taken;
          (2) the measurement of the actual level of the services rendered plus the efforts to modify, when necessary, the provision of these services in the light of the results of the measurement.

Quality audit   a systematic and independent examination of the effectiveness of the quality system or of its parts.

Quality characteristic
          some property of the product or service that contributes to its quality.

Quality circle   a process whereby staff at every layer in an organisation work together as a team to improve quality of service or life.

Relevance   services provided are applicable to the needs of the client.

Reliable   (1) operates a system which is cost-effective, efficient and dependable;
          (2) depend upon with confidence.
          (3) of measurement - produces consistent results.

Resourced   has all the appropriate resources to operate.

Resourceful	copes despite lack of resources.
Respected	has skills/personality admired by others.
Responsibility	the obligation that an individual assumes when undertaking to carry out delegated functions. The individual who authorises the delegated function retains accountability.
Standard	(1) an accepted or approved example or statement of something against which measurement and/or judgement takes place; a level of quality relevant to the activity; (2) a statement which defines agreed objectives for the level of excellence, and describes the skills, resources or results required to achieve the level of excellence in terms which can be used to measure achievement; 'The desired and achievable level of performance corresponding with a criterion or criteria against which actual performance is compared.' Castledine (1983)
Structure	the characteristics of the providers of care, of the tools and resources at their disposal, and of the physical and organisational settings in which they work.
Valid	of measurement—measuring what is intended should be measured.
Value	a personal moral or ethical principle which forms the basis of individuals' determination of their standards.

USEFUL READING

Acheson D 1987 Assuring quality. British Journal of Occupational Therapy 50(7):247-248

Bromley A I 1978 The patient care audit. Physiotherapy 64(9):270-271

Bromley I, Sutcliffe B, Hunter A 1987 Physiotherapy services: a basis for development of standards. King's Fund, London

Carr-Hill R, Dalley G 1991 Quality management initiatives in the NHS: booklets 1-4. Centre for Health Economics, University of York, York

Chartered Society of Physiotherapy 1990 Standards of physiotherapy practice. Chartered Society of Physiotherapy, London

College of Occupational Therapists 1989-1991 Standards, policies and proceedings: documents. College of Occupational Therapy, London

COT 1990 Contracting for quality. British Journal of Occupational Therapy 53(2):83-84

Crawford M   1989 Setting standards in occupational therapy. British Journal of Occupational Therapy 52(8):294-297

CSP Discussion Document 1988 The practice of physiotherapy. Physiotherapy 74(8)

Department of Health 1989 A strategy for nursing. Department of Health, Nursing Division, London

Di Primio A 1987 Quality assurance in service organisations. Chilton, Radnor

Dixon P, Carr-Hill R 1989 The NHS and its customers: booklet 2, customer feedback surveys—an introduction to survey methods. Centre for Health Economics, University of York, York

Donabedian A 1980 The definition of quality and approaches to its assessment. Health Administration Press, Ann Arbor

Donabedian A 1985 Twenty years of research on the quality of medical care. Evaluation and the Health Professions 8(3):243-265

Ellis R (ed) 1988 Professional competence and quality assurance in the caring professions. Croom Helm, Beckenham

Garvin D A 1988 Managing quality: the strategic and competitive edge. Collier Macmillan, New York

Goldstone L 1987 Quality counts in nursing. Newcastle-Upon-Tyne Polytechnic, Newcastle-Upon-Tyne

Greene J, D'Oliveira M 1982 Learning to use statistical tests in psychology. Open University Press, Milton Keynes

Grimmer K 1989 Quality assurance: an integral part of private physiotherapy practice. Australian Journal of Physiotherapy 35(3):189-190

Heath J R 1978 Problem oriented medical systems. Physiotherapy 64(9):269-270

High D 1988 Management of quality. The Institute of Health Services Management, London

Hinkle D, Wiersma W, Jurs S G 1982 Basic behavioral statistics. Houghton Mifflin, Boston

Hutchins D 1990 In pursuit of quality. Pitman, London

Jacobs K 1989 Functions of a manager in occupational therapy. Slack, New Jersey

Kemp N, Richardson E 1990 Quality assurance in nursing practice. Butterworth Heinemann, London

Kitson A, Harvey G 1991 Bibliography of nursing quality assurance and standards of care. Scutari Press, London

Kitson A L, Hyndman S J, Harvey G, Yerrell P 1990 Quality patient care, an introduction to RCN dynamic standard setting system (DySSSy). Scutari Press, London

Klein R 1983 The politics of the National Health Service. Longman, London

Lang N, Clinton J 1984 Assessment of quality of nursing care. In: Werley H, Fitzpatrick J (eds) Annual review of nursing research, Vol II. Springer, New York

Law M, Ryan B, Townsend E, O'Shea B 1989 Criteria mapping: a method of quality assurance. The American Journal of Occupational Therapy 43(2):104-109

McColl M, Quinn B 1985 A quality assurance method for community occupational therapy. The American Journal of Occupational Therapy 39(9):570-577

McCulloch D 1991 Can we measure output?—quality adjusted life years, health indices and occupational therapy. British Journal of Occupational Therapy 54(6):219-221

Mead J 1989 Setting standards in physiotherapy. Physiotherapy 75(3):183-184

Murphy C S 1987 Clinical audit: measuring the quality of individual clinical performance. British Journal of Occupational Therapy 50(3):83-85

Oppenheim A N 1986 Questionnaire design and attitude measurement. Gower, Aldershot

Palmer R H, Donabedian A, Povar G J 1991 Striving for quality in health care. Health Administration Press, Ann Arbor

Pearson A (ed) 1987 Nursing quality measurement: quality assurance methods for peer review. John Wiley, Chichester

Ratcliff Hill J 1977 Problem-oriented approach to physical therapy care. American Physical Therapy Association

Redfern S J, Norman I J 1990 Measuring the quality of nursing care: a consideration of different approaches. Journal of Advanced Nursing 15:1260-1271

Sale D 1990 Quality assurance. Macmillan, London

Shaw C D 1980 Aspects of audit 1-5. British Medical Journal 280(6226-6230) May-June

Shaw C D 1986 Time to close up the quality gap. Health and Social Service Journal, Jan 23rd, p110

Shaw C D 1989 Medical audit. King's Fund, London

Shaw C D 1990 How the doctors do it. Nursing Standard 5(3):52-53

Stricker F, Rodriguez A 1988 Handbook of quality assurance in mental health. Plenum, New York

Willis L D, Linwood M E 1984 Measuring the quality of care. Churchill Livingstone, Edinburgh

Wilson C R M 1987 Hospital wide quality assurance: models for implementation and development. Saunders, Toronto

REFERENCES

Argyle M 1969 Social interaction. Methuen, London

Australian Nurses Journal 1982 Glossary of terms in Q.A. 11(7):18-20

British Standards Institution 1987 BS5750 part 0, sections 0.1 and 0.2:1987 (ISO 9000 - 1987). British Standard Institution, Milton Keynes

Carr-Hill R, Dalley G 1991 Quality management initiatives in the NHS: booklets 1-4. Centre for Health Economics, University of York, York

Castledine G 1983 In the best possible care. Nursing Mirror 156(19):22

Chartered Society of Physiotherapy 1990 Standards of physiotherapy practice. Chartered Society of Physiotherapy, London

College of Occupational Therapists Educational Department 1987 Study day on quality assurance. British Journal of Occupational Therapy 50(7):234-236

College of Occupational Therapists 1989-1991 Standards, policies and proceedings: documents. College of Occupational Therapy, London

Crawford M 1989 Definitions relating to quality assurance. British Journal of Occupational Therapy 52(7):270

Daugherty J, Mason E 1987 Excelcare. Price Waterhouse, Bristol

Department of Health 1990 The quality of medical care: report of the Standing Medical Advisory Committee. HMSO, London

DOH 1989 Working for Patients, CMND.555 . HMSO, London

DOH 1989 Working for patients, medical audit, working paper no. 6. HMSO, London

Donabedian A 1966 Evaluating the quality of medical care. Milbank Memorial Fund Quarterly 44(2):166-206

Editorial 1990 Multi-therapy audit study. Therapy 16(41):1

Editorial 1990 COT to measure standards. Therapy 16(37):3

Ellis M 1987 Quality: who cares? (the Casson memorial lecture). British Journal of Occupational Therapy 50(6):195-200

European Newsletter on Quality Assurance 1984 Ten on terminology. CBO, Utrecht, 1(2):2 and 2(1):2

Feigenbaum A V 1961 Total quality control. McGraw-Hill, New York

Garvin D A 1988 Managing quality: the strategic and competitive edge. Collier Macmillan, New York

Goldstone L A, Ball J A, Collier M M 1983 Monitor, an index of the quality of nursing care for acute medical and surgical wards. Newcastle-Upon-Tyne Polytechnic, Newcastle-Upon-Tyne

Hofer J (ed) 1989 Glossary of terms used in the management of quality, 6th edn. European Organisation for Quality

Hyde P 1984 Quality circles: something for everyone. Nursing Times 80(48):49-50

Juran J M (ed) 1988 Juran's quality control handbook, 4th edn. McGraw-Hill, New York, section 9 quality assurance and section 33 service industries

Kitson A L, Hyndman S J, Harvey G, Yerrell P 1990 Quality patient care, an introduction to RCN dynamic standard setting system (DySSSy). Scutari Press, London

Kitson A L, Kendall H 1986 Quality assurance. Nursing Times 82(35):28-31

Lang N, Clinton J 1984 Assessment of quality of nursing care. In: Werley H, Fitzpatrick J (eds) Annual review of nursing research, Vol II. Springer, New York

Maxwell R J 1984 Quality assessment in health. British Medical Journal, 288:1470-1471

Mayers M, Norby R B, Watson A B 1977 Quality assurance for patient care: nursing perspectives. Appleton-Century-Crofts, New York

Nichol D K 1989 Quality in the NHS: letter el(89)/mb/114 from Duncan Nichol, Chief Executive of NHS Management Executive to the Chairmen and General Managers of Health Authorities. Department of Health Press Office, London

Rooney E M 1988 A proposed quality system specification for the National Health Service. Quality Assurance 14(2):45-53

Royal College of Nursing 1989 A framework for quality, RCN standards of care project. Royal College of Nursing, London

Royal College of Nursing 1990 The dynamic standard setting system. Royal College of Nursing, London

Sanazaro P J 1986 The principle of quality assurance in health care. World Hospitals xxii(1):27-28

Schroeder P S, Maibusch R M 1984 Nursing quality assurance: a unit based approach. Aspen, Maryland

Schroeder et al 1986 In: Giebing H 1986 Nursing quality assurance. European Newsletter on Quality Assurance 3(2):5

Shaw C D 1986 Introducing quality assurance paper no 64. King's Fund, London

Stebbing L 1990 Quality management in the service industry. Ellis Horwood, Chichester

Van Maanen H M 1979 Improvement of quality of nursing care: a goal to challenge in the 1980's. Journal of Advanced Nursing 6:3-9

Wandelt M, Ager J 1974 Quality patient care scale (QualPaCS).
Appleton-Century-Crofts, New York

Weed L L 1971 The problem-oriented record as a basic tool in medical education, patient care and clinical research. Annals of Clinical Research 3:131-134

Wheeler N 1989 Occupational therapy and cost effectiveness. Health Care Management 4(3):22-24

W.H.O. 1982 Quality assurance of health services. WHO, Copenhagen